Activities

for the Elderly

Volume 2

A Guide to Working
with Residents
with Significant
Physical
and Cognitive
Disabilities

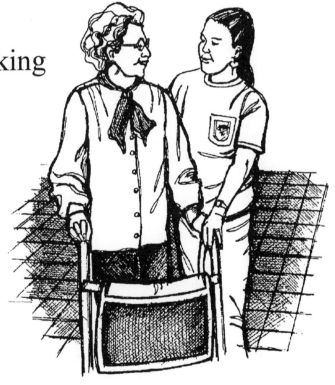

Sandra D. Parker
Carol Will

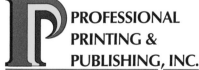

PP **PROFESSIONAL**
PRINTING &
PUBLISHING, INC.

P.O. Box 5758 · Bossier City, LA 71171-5758
318-746-6880 · 1-800-551-8783 · FAX 318-746-6995
Web Site: http://www.ppandp.com · E-mail: order@ppandp.com

Published by

Idyll Arbor, Inc.

PO Box 720, Ravensdale, WA 98051 (425) 432-3231

© 1993 Idyll Arbor, Inc.

Printed in the United States of America

First Printing 1993
Second Printing 1995
Third Printing 1998

Cover Design: Original Photography: Sarah Blaschko
                  Original Drawing: Linda Anderson

ISBN 1-882883-01-2

Table of Contents

Chapter 1

Introduction

Those of us who serve seniors have made great strides in caring for their bodies and the physical environment. We have rules and regulations that govern residential and long-term care facilities. We have established programs to help care for elders in their homes. We are gaining knowledge to help older people live longer, in better health and in more comfort through their declining years. Time has come to explore the *quality* of life in old age. With declining function (either physical or cognitive) many of our elderly question the purpose and meaning in their lives.

In ages past, most people who suffered acute illness or accidents died fairly quickly. Today we have conquered many of the acute illnesses and can often prevent death from accidents. This leaves us with a two-fold problem: 1) many victims of accidents are left with severe functional limitations, and 2) people who are older have more chronic conditions (both physical and cognitive) that limit their ability to participate in "normal" activities.

Activities are very important in maintaining quality of life which includes independence, enjoyment, physical, cognitive, and emotional fitness. In addition, participating in activities tends to give us the chance to engage in socialization and to help others. Preparing and presenting activities for elderly who are well or even many elderly who are ill is rewarding and usually straight forward. Those folks can tell us what interests them and what they are able to do. They enjoy sharing past experiences that help us to plan activities relating to their past and which are meaningful for them.

Activity planning becomes more difficult when the people with whom we are working are not able to communicate or participate in the usual activities. Yet, we recognize the importance of involving these people in activities. Organizations and agencies who regulate and monitor long-term care facilities also recognize the importance of meaningful activities in maintaining quality of life. There is increasing emphasis from survey teams concerning activities for the adults who are low-functioning—emphasis for activities that reflect life-long interests of the adults and on activities that will have meaning for them.

In conversations with activity staff, long-term care administrators and families, we found a hunger for information on activities for adults who are low functioning. A search for written resources of activities reveals few references specific to the topic. It is our hope that this book will fill that need.

This book is intended to help find interesting and meaningful activities for the adults who are low functioning whether they are in long-term care facilities or at home. It is our hope that the information we present will help not only activity directors, but other long-term care workers, volunteers and family members to provide a higher quality of life for the adults in their care.

Who Is "Low Functioning"?

In conversations with activity staff, each seems to have a slightly different definition of "low-functioning." In the general older adult population functioning levels are described as follows:

1) High to Moderate Functioning—independent, able to do own personal care. This includes:

- Activities of daily living—bathing, dressing, tolleting, transferring, controlling waste, and feeding self
- Instrumental activities of daily living—able to use the telephone, shop, prepare meals, do housekeeping, do laundry, travel independently (either drive self or use public transportation), take own medications and handle finances.
- Cognitive abilities—able to express values and goals, able to communicate and understand information, make decisions, understand actions taken, take care of personal property and assets, recognize and understand relationships with others, demonstrate emotional stability and show reasonable long and short term memory.

In general, these adults have adequate vision and hearing, minimal chronic disease and are active physically and socially.

2) Low functioning—those older adults who for any reason cannot completely care for themselves. Help in one or all of the above areas is required for survival.

When one considers the residents in long-term care facilities or those cared for in the home on a full time basis, they all could be considered "low-functioning" in terms of the general population. All need help to survive. Hence we need to define low-functioning as it applies in home care or long-term care situations.

Generally (in terms of activities) low-functioning would include those who are very limited physically or cognitively and are unlikely to improve. This would include those with dementia, with severe arthritis, with a stroke with extensive paralysis, with multiple amputations, or, in other words, those who require staff assistance for most or all activities of daily living. Those with highly impaired vision or hearing might also qualify if the losses are recent. Those with long-term losses have usually made adequate adjustments, hence their impairment does not normally interfere with functioning.

The most difficult limitation for most activity staff to deal with is cognitive impairment. Cognitive impairment may be due to Alzheimer's or related disorders or to reversible conditions such as mental illness or depression. Many times these people appear normal physically, but are unable to function in normal activities because of limited understanding, inappropriate interactions with others, withdrawn behavior, or other cognitive reasons. They simply cannot or will not participate in normal activities.

Whatever the cause, planning and implementing activities for these adults is a challenge!

Memory

Research indicates that there are two main types of memories. Declarative memory stores facts while procedural memory enables us to learn and perform tasks and skills. Most of us use both types of memory at the same time. However, declarative (fact) memory can be affected by injury or disease while procedural (skills) memory still functions. This explains why a person with dementia might not remember his/her name, but will still be able to read signs—even if s/he does not understand what the sign says.

The cognitive activity involved in the process of storage and retrieval of information is extremely complex. Memories are stored in several places in the brain and the more that memory is used the stronger the storage network becomes. This is called long-term memory.

Short term memory is for new information. That information is stored in short term memory until we decide if it is important enough to store in long-term memory. When we are young we store many things in long-term memory. As we age, we become more selective—we only store things that are relevant and have meaning to us.

In dementia of the Alzheimer's type, the brain cells that process and store short-term memory are slowly destroyed. The individual with dementia is unable to store new information. Old memories remain much longer. The more important those memories are, the longer they are remembered.

The resident with Alzheimer's also has slower brain function. It is very important to give the person extra time to process what you have said before you expect a response. The resident may not recognize you even though you were just in the room or see him/her every day. His/her days are full of new experiences and people!

Before We Start

Childhood, youth, early adulthood, middle age, old age. All are important phases of our lives. Our families change as we age, as do our roles in life—child, sibling, spouse, parent, grandparent. As we near the end of life we look back at those roles with varying emotions. Memories of good times and bad times become important as we search for meaning in our lives.

The adult who is low functioning may lose recent memories and not be able to relate to recent roles, but may remember, and indeed seem to be living, in the past. For instance; the resident may not recognize a son or daughter as his/her child. The son or daughter may remind the resident of his/her brother or sister and s/he may call the children by the sibling's name. By using activities that reflect the past, you are approaching the individual in his/her present.

The success of your activities will depend, to a certain extent, on conditions surrounding the individual's formative years:

- World, regional and local events
- The area of the country where the individual grew up
- The ethnic background of the family and neighborhood
- Social standing of the family
- Economic conditions of the region, neighborhood and family

- Work ethic of the family and social group
- Moral or religious values of the family and social group
- Accepted recreational activities of the time

While it may be impossible to find specific information about the family, an understanding of the cultural values of the time, ethnic background, religious values, and recreational activities will help make your activities meaningful to the adult who is low functioning.

Some activities are appropriate for anyone within a certain age group or with similar backgrounds. For instance, sing-a-longs using songs from the twenties are appropriate for people who were young adults in the twenties. Watercolor classes may appeal to those with artistic interests. Travelogues are enjoyed by people who are curious about the sights and sounds of the world. Reading or writing groups appeal to the intellectually curious.

The activity professional knows the events and interests from each era represented by his or her residents. World events, music, entertainment or games, occupations, family roles, all make an impact—especially during teen and young adult years. By planning activities that represent those times, the activity professional appeals to the residents and indicates an interest in them (validates them) as important people.

Activity histories, taken for planning purposes, help to determine common interests of residents or patients receiving home care. When planning for adults who are low functioning, life and activity histories become even more important because the present often is painful or recent memory is impaired, making the past more real or meaningful. In long term care facilities activity histories must be part of the admission process. The same information can be helpful when planning for individuals at home.

First you need to find out all you can about the person, Age, place of birth, education, marital and family history, provide a basic view of the person. Life style history will further define the person. Occupation and hobbies, church and organizational affiliation, travel experience, etc. will give you guidelines for activities. You will want to know his/her normal schedule and activity participation (past and present). Was this person a participant or spectator? Leader or follower? Did s/he enjoy active or passive activities?

People who share a particular event or time in history are called cohorts. This means that they have shared experiences that influence the way they perceive the world. One way to classify cohorts is by the time in history in which they reached maturity. There are some events and interests that these groups of people share.

Events and Interests by Era

People born Before 1920

Born before nuclear energy, TV, or computers, grew up in the depression
- These folks are frugal
- They do not spend money easily—even when the have it
- They did not grow up with regular health care
- Families were closed units—what went on within the family stayed there
- They learned well-defined sex or gender roles
- The entertainment was inexpensive, often within family or church group
- Music was generally sentimental and optimistic with references to work, hardships, and love
- Games were non-electronic and often homemade—bingo, checkers, cribbage, etc.

People Born Between 1920 and 1925

Biggest impact was World War II
- For many their identity and status was gained through some mode of participation in World War II (served in armed forces, used ration coupons, worked in war industry, etc.)
- The work force expanded to include women
- There was an increase in regular health and dental care
- Education and housing programs were available for veterans
- Housing was very inexpensive
- Music was patriotic and nonsensical
- Entertainment centered around movies and radio

People Born Between 1926 and 1940

Grew up in an era of rapidly increasing earnings and heavy spending
- They had better pension plans and medical benefits
- They became used to going to professionals for services
- In later years they become aware of wellness

- Families became scattered and there was an increased incidence of divorce
- Entertainment included television, stereo, and VCR
- Music ranged from romantic to rock and roll

Second you need to find out the person's present condition, abilities, and treatment schedule. The diagnosis will help to determine activity level and probable improvement or deterioration of condition. Coping with illness requires a lot of energy. Consider the amount of energy available for activities. The types of impairments and the degree to which the person can overcome them is important. Knowing what treatments are prescribed and the schedule for those treatments will help you know how much free time the person has.

Finally, how much are family and friends involved with the resident? One reason adults who are impaired have few visitors is that family or friends are uncomfortable visiting because they don't know what to say or do when they visit. Families and friends may welcome the opportunity to help with specific activities.

Finding all of the above information may take some detective work. The resident or patient receiving in-home care may be able to give you information verbally, but frequently are not able to communicate in that manner. You may find some physical clues such as skin that has obviously been exposed to the sun—indicating an outdoor person, or smooth hands that might indicate that the person has not performed a lot of manual labor. Verbal clues such as a foreign accent or language usage may be helpful.

The family can be very helpful as they are most likely to have knowledge about recent activity level and schedules. They can fill in personal history. Friends often have insights into individuals that others do not have. They often know more about interests, likes and dislikes, loves and hates, than even family members.

Use all the resources available to become acquainted with the adult who is impaired. Only then will you be able to plan activities that will reflect his/her interests giving you a greater chance of sparking interest and involving the person.

Successful activities also require planning of environmental factors. The room should be just large enough for the activity to help focus on the activity and prevent wandering. Bright colors, comfortable furniture, adequate non-glare lighting, non-glare flooring with a solid pattern, and noise control, contribute to an optimal atmosphere.

Small groups of people with similar functional levels are easier to work with. Adequate help is essential for successful activities.

Keep equipment simple, using as few items as possible. Have only essential items present, but make sure you have everything you will need for the activity.

Activities are an important part of the day for the resident or person receiving in-home care. The activity professional needs to coordinate with nursing and therapy routines so the resident will be as alert as possible with adequate energy for activities. Many people prefer mornings for activities although late afternoon activities could help with sun downing (agitation late in the afternoon or early evening) problems. Physical activities might be scheduled at a time when the individual needs a physical outlet to release pent-up energy. Alternate active and passive activities and remember to schedule rest times. Consult with caregivers to find the times when the individual is most alert. Schedule around that time for optimal benefits from activities.

Measuring "Family Health" and Involvement

The Family APGAR (Smilkstein, 1978) is an easy to use, quick method to measure the degree of family sharing and involvement. The activity director reads each statement and then "rates" each resident's situation using a "0" (zero) for "almost always", "1" for "some of the time", and "2" for "hardly ever." After reading all five statements and adding up the score, the activity director will have the resident's Family APGAR score. Scores over 3 (out of a possible 10) are considered a problem. Those residents with a score of 5 or more may be good candidates for extra volunteer and staff time.

Family APGAR Scale

The Family APGAR is a screening tool to help the activity director determine if the resident needs extra staff or volunteer time. Read each statement and then determine a score by using "0" (zero) for "almost always", "1" for "some of the time", and "2" for "hardly ever." Scores over 3 (out of a possible 10) are considered a problem. Residents with a score of 5 or more may be good candidates for extra volunteer and/or staff time.

Adaptation
1. In my family we help each other out. If we can't find the help we need within the family, we have places and people in the community to help.

Partnership
2. In my family we make decisions by talking things out and then reaching an agreement.

Growth
3. In my family we help each other achieve our desires and support each other so that we can grow and change.

Affection
4. In my family we are able to share all kinds of feelings with each other including love, anger, and sorrow.

Resolve
5. In my family we share what we have including our time, our space, and our money.

Note: If some of the residents do not have family close by but have a good support network of friends, use the Family APGAR using the statement "My friends and I" instead of "In my family we."

The Family APGAR way developed by Smilkstein in 1978.

Chapter 2

Activity Categories and Benefits

When planning activities, it is important to be aware of the various categories of activities so you will have a well-rounded program. There are several different sources of activity categories. The United States Government requires activities that meet the residents' needs, no matter how well or disabled they are. These needs are defined as a continuum, from the most able ("empowerment") to the least able ("supportive") to help himself/herself. A definition of the three levels is listed below.

Hierarchy of Activities

Activities that promote increased self-respect by providing opportunities for self-expression, personal responsibility, and choice. Examples might include: arts classes, drama group, gardening, discussion groups, autobiography development, opportunities for volunteering, involvement in Resident Councils, etc. (Empowerment Activities).

Activities that promote physical, cognitive, social, and emotional health. Examples might include: exercise programs, competitive games, spelling bees, puzzles, dances and parties, religious programs, relaxation programs, etc. (Maintenance Activities).

Activities that provide stimulation or solace to residents who cannot generally benefit from either maintenance or empowerment activities. Examples might include: sensory stimulation activities such as colorful mobile objects, familiar music, familiar odors, familiar tastes, touching with different textures, hand massage, or body movement (perhaps assisted). Other examples include reading, or talking with the person about his or her life (family, occupation, hobbies, etc.). (Supportive Activities).

No matter how abled or disabled the resident is, s/he will have some definite preferences for the types of activities that s/he enjoys. Activities and leisure interests can be divided into eight categories. The resident will most likely have a preference for one or two types of activities and a dislike for one or two types of activities. The activity director will find it

11

easier to accomplish empowerment, maintenance, and to be supportive of the resident if s/he knows the resident's preferences. The eight types of activities are listed below.

Eight Types of Activities

1. **Physical Activities** that provide opportunities for increasing or maintaining physical strength, endurance, coordination, and range of motion.

2. **Outdoor Activities** that allow the individual to enjoy the sights, sounds, and events that are available when one is outside and which provide a connection with natural cycles of life.

3. **Mechanical Activities** which involve the building, fixing, or making things run.

4. **Artistic Activities** which allow the individual to express his/her creative use of materials or words.

5. **Service Activities** which allow the individual to help others, thereby increasing his/her self-esteem and feelings of usefulness.

6. **Social Activities** which allows the individual to interact with other people.

7. **Cultural Activities** which allows the individual to appreciate someone else's expression of artistic skill.

8. **Reading Activities** which entertain or inform through the use of printed word or stories on tape.

There are several important benefits that residents or patients in home care receive from activities no matter what type of activity they are engaged in. These benefits are usually grouped together into what are called "domains." For the purpose of this book we have divided the benefits of all the activities listed into one of five domains. The domains are physical, cognitive, emotional, social, and spiritual.

Domains of Activities

Physical Activities can help maintain or increase physical strength and endurance. This helps to maintain muscle tone, increases cardiac functioning, respiratory capacity, coordination and range of motion. They also help relieve tension, resulting in relaxation.

Cognitive Activities which stimulate the cognitive processes, improving concentration and problem solving, and help to retain language, interpersonal and memory skills.

Emotional Activities provide opportunity for enjoyment, laughter, expressions of sadness, anger, competition and satisfaction.

Spiritual Activities provide opportunity to expand spiritually. One can review his/her life in terms of values and find meaning and a purpose for being. One can feel a connection with one's self, others and the universe.

Social Activities provide an opportunity for social interaction, enhance communication and help one to develop a sense of belonging.

These benefits are important to everyone regardless of his/her functioning level. We must strive to provide activities that benefit those who are physically or cognitively impaired as well as those who are able to participate and respond.

Many activities can be adapted to correspond to the functioning level of your resident. Group activities such as exercise class will work well if you keep the group small, simplify and slow the pace and limit the time to correspond with attention spans.

Individual activities may be more appropriate for the person who is roombound, has no verbal response, who is removed from reality, extremely disoriented or withdrawn, disruptive, or who becomes agitated in group situations.

It is important to participate with the individual who is low functioning and show him/her that you appreciate sharing time together. The adult who is low functioning spends most of the time <u>receiving</u> care from others. We cannot stress enough how valuable it is to allow the individual the opportunity to <u>give</u>. Spend time interacting with the individual and show appreciation of that time spent together.

General rules to remember in adapting activities for individuals who are low-functioning:

- Keep it simple.
- Provide an example.
- Give one direction at a time.
- Give time for understanding.
- Keep sessions short.
- Provide opportunity for success.

Chapter 3

Involving Others

Providing activities for the adult who is low functioning can be a time consuming task. Most activities require small groups or individual attention. Limited participation on the part of the resident means more work for the provider. Your time may be very limited—scheduling, paperwork, organizational details, plus a full activity schedule all of which require excellent time management skills.

One way to make the most of your time and skills is to involve others in providing actual activities. With proper training and documentation, volunteers, family members and even other staff members can enhance your activity program. The time spent in preparation will pay huge dividends in an efficient, yet excellent program.

Volunteers

The first step in utilizing volunteers to work with adults who are low functioning is the selection process. Through interviews you should be able to determine if the potential volunteer has the patience and commitment to work with this group. Patience is a very important attribute since the volunteer will have to repeat simple instructions, wait for response, and resist an urge to help the resident. Sometimes there will be no response at all, thus no outward recognition of what the volunteer is attempting to do. You will have to assure the volunteer that his/her involvement is worthwhile and meaningful.

The second step is training. A basic understanding of the conditions that result in low functioning will give the volunteer an understanding of limitations and expectations. If you do not feel comfortable doing this, perhaps someone else from the nursing or therapy staff can provide this part of the training. The volunteer should be given an understanding of the categories and benefits of activities so s/he can appreciate the value of his/her work. It will also help the volunteer if s/he has the opportunity to observe and question activity staff working with the adult who is low functioning.

The third step is providing tasks. Volunteers appreciate clear instructions of their assignments. By giving them detailed activity plans such as those presented in this book, you will help make their visits successful.

Finally, remember evaluation! Give your volunteers feedback frequently. Praise them when appropriate and learn the fine art of constructive criticism when things are not going so well. *Remember their only paycheck is your token of appreciation.* Evaluation also applies to your volunteer program. Set goals for your program and schedule regular evaluation of the status of those goals.

Family Members and Friends

Involving family members and friends in your activity plan accomplishes three purposes. First, it extends your activity program. Second, it allows family and friends to be useful and feel needed. Third, it fosters the relationship between the resident and family and/or friends.

When we talk with many of the families and friends of residents living in nursing homes and of patients receiving in-home care, they express frustration about visiting their loved one. They don't know what to say or what to do. This discomfort results in fewer and increasingly shorter visits. Others become overly concerned about the care their loved one is receiving and can become disruptive to the staff and other residents.

During your initial interview with the family, you can enlist their aid in helping with your activity goals for the resident, Families can participate in groups with the resident. The resident may feel more comfortable when a family member is present. Families are especially helpful in one-on-one activities. As with volunteers, training and written activity plans are very important. You can work out documentation details with the aid of a flow sheet that is simple and convenient for the family.

Staff

Staff members are involved in many activities with residents. With some orientation and cooperation, they could provide therapeutic activities. Nurses aides for example, could discuss current events while bathing or making beds. Housekeeping personnel might help change the tapes in the resident's tape player or VCR while they clean the resident's room. Once again training and documentation is vital to success.

Administrative support is necessary. You should explore the idea in a staff inservice. Ask the staff for ideas. Once they understand your goals and purpose, they will share their ideas for activities that will expand your program. Again, keep documentation simple and easy but be sure to document!

All this takes organizational skills. You must be able to train, then delegate to your helpers. With today's budget constraints, using volunteers (from outside, families, or staff) is imperative for an effective activity program for the adult who is low functioning.

Chapter 4

How to Use This Book

The following activity plans are intended to be used as guidelines for professionals and for volunteers. The activity plans are designed to be used independently, Each plan gives the time recommended for the activity, the desired environment, the materials needed, the benefits expected from the activity, the activity description and the conversation starters (questions designed to encourage the individual to converse). Individual activity plans may be given to volunteers or family, with all benefits and instructions readily available for their information.

Remember when you are doing these activities that some of them may bring out negative instead of positive reactions from the resident. If the person becomes agitated, frustrated, or is unable to cope with stresses associated with the activity, you should stop the activity. If the activity brings out feelings of sadness or loss *and* you can help the resident deal with those feelings, the activity is succeeding and should be continued. Happiness, feelings of accomplishment, and contentment are examples of positive benefits from these activities. Dealing with negative feelings and getting on with life is positive, too. However, you should stop the activity and try something else when an activity doesn't succeed.

The materials needed for the activities can usually be obtained easily with little or no expense. We encourage use of available materials. We have found that service groups such as church groups or organizational auxiliaries are willing to help gather materials. Again, your creativity will suggest alternatives for the recommended materials that will not only suffice but will enhance the activity.

Activities should reflect the interests of the individual. Therefore the activities in chapters five through eleven are grouped under interest topics. Chapters twelve through fourteen contain activities that are not specific for any interest, but are in categories necessary for a well-rounded program. The individual's activity history will indicate which are appropriate for him/her.

Planning activities for the adult who is low functioning is challenging, but rewarding. Remember to have fun!

Chapter 5

Family Roles

This group of activities focuses on the many roles an individual plays in his/her family. We all begin as dependent children, but soon our roles differ. Roles may include brother or sister, cousin, husband or wife, parent, aunt or uncle, grand parent, etc. Roles also differ according to the size of the family, number of generations in the household, health of family members, etc.

We need to remember that a person's role may not have been a happy one. The individual may not have wanted that role or may even have resented the role. Those feelings may come to the surface during activities which focus on family roles. Most of the memories, however, will be pleasant and positive.

The activities in this chapter are intended to bring back memories of childhood through adulthood. We have tried to include activities that utilize all the senses. You will think of other ways to add to these activities. Let our ideas inspire your imagination!

Family Photos

Group Size	One on one
Time	10 to 20 minutes
Environment	Quiet room
Materials	Resident family photos
	Staff family photos
	Family photos from magazines

Benefits

cognitive: describing past knowledge, identifying, remembering relatives from the past

spiritual: exploring the continuation of life and one's place in that continuum

emotional: enjoyment, perhaps expression of sadness and loss, security, love, happiness

social: interacting with others

Activity

- Lay photos out on a table and ask the resident to identify the people pictured.
- Ask questions about each person. What relation are they to you? What do you remember most about him/her? Did this person make you laugh? Cry? What things did you do together?

Conversation Starters

- Let the resident choose from two photos.
- Show photos of your family. Talk about the questions above.
- Show photos from magazines that picture families. Speculate about how that family feels about each other, what they like to do together, etc.

School Reminiscence

Group Size	One on one
Time	10 to 15 minutes
Environment	Quiet area with table and chairs
Materials	Blackboard, chalk and erasers
	Ruler, pen, pencil, tablet
	Inkwell
	Old school books, flash cards

Benefits

cognitive: describing past events, labeling, explaining, calculating, estimating

physical: fine motor manipulation, dexterity, eye-hand coordination

emotional: enjoyment, expression of feelings associated with school days, (satisfaction, frustration, worry, excitement, self-doubt, shyness, pride)

social: interacting with objects, interacting with others

Activity

- Allow the resident to handle and use the school items one at a time. Encourage him/her to talk about school including:
  - size of school
  - best friends
  - favorite teachers
- Encourage him/her to do simple penmanship exercises, math exercises, and reading.

Conversation Starters

- Do you remember who was the "teacher's pet"? What privileges did that person have?
- Do you remember the sound of chalk squeaking on the blackboard? What other sounds do you remember from your school days?
- Can you describe your desk? Did it have an inkwell?
- What was your favorite subject?
- What extracurricular activities did you participate in?

Songs from Childhood

Group Size	One on one or small group
Time	5 to 20 minutes
Environment	Small area such as music room with no distractions. Comfortable, upright chairs.
Materials	No materials necessary. Optional materials: Piano or other musical instrument Words to children's songs (large print)

Benefits

cognitive: reproducing past known combination of words, turning words into actions

physical: creates opportunity for deeper breathing, non-locomotor movement

emotional: joy, laughter, pleasure

social: interacting with others

spiritual: reminder of basis of values

Activity

- Come to the activity with four or five children's songs in mind. Be familiar with the actions involved.
- Suggestions: Mary Had a Little Lamb; Three Blind Mice; Row, Row, Row Your Boat; I'm a Little Teapot; Itsy Bitsy Spider
- Sing through the song once then ask the resident to join you. Encourage use of motions.
- For the resident who is less responsive—gently move the resident's arms or hands as you sing.
- Ask the resident to suggest songs. Encourage him/her to teach you songs.

Conversation Starters

- Do you remember singing songs when you were a child?
- What was your favorite song?
- Who did you sing with?
- Was music a part of your family activities?

- Did you sing songs with your children? Grandchildren?
- Were they the same songs you sang as a child?

Childhood Fashions

Group Size	One on one activity
Time	10 to 15 minutes
Environment	Quiet area with comfortable furniture
Materials	Children's clothing from the time of the person's childhood (may be obtained from family, second hand store, antique dealer, or museum). May include: christening dress, knickers, girls dress, high top shoes, suspenders, cap or sun bonnet

Benefits

cognitive: describing, identifying, naming, explaining, giving examples, relating

emotional: enjoyment, satisfaction, happiness, sadness

spiritual: memories of religious significance

social: interacting with objects, interacting with others, concept of self

Activity

- Show the resident articles of children's clothing. Allow him/her to touch and smell. Encourage the resident to tell stories that the clothing brings to mind. Discuss the items of clothing in terms of the resident's childhood and of his/her children's childhood.
- If the resident is unresponsive, relate stories you have heard about the resident's childhood and/or talk about your own experiences.

Conversation Starters

- Did your family have any special clothing that was saved for use by all the children in the family (i.e., christening dress)?
- Did you have a favorite clothes? Tell me about it.
- Did you wear hand-me-downs? How did you feel about them?
- What type of shoes (pants, underwear, dress, hat) did you wear?
- How many shoes (pants, dresses, etc.) did you have?

Toys of Childhood

Group Size	One on one activity
Time	15 to 20 minutes
Environment	Quiet area with comfortable chairs and table
Materials	Assortment of old toys (may come from family, antique or second hand store, museum, or private collection): tops, wooden cars and trucks, old trains, farm toys, Lincoln Logs, dolls, doll dishes, paper dolls, marbles, jacks

Benefits

cognitive: describing past knowledge, stating, demonstrating, long term memory retention, concentrating

physical: fine motor functioning (finger manipulation)

emotional: enjoyment, laughter, curiosity, joy, happiness, enthusiasm, contentment

social: interacting with objects, interacting with others, concept of self

Activity

Show the resident one toy at a time and encourage him/her to play with it. Discuss how the toy was made and how it was used.

Conversation Starters

- Did you ever play with any toys like these?
- Tell me about your favorite toy.
- Did you fight with other children about toys? Who did you usually play with most?
- Did you make your own toys? Did you make toys for gifts?
- Do you remember toys you gave your children? Tell me about some of them.

Childhood Chores

Group Size	One on one
Time	10 to 15 minutes
Environment	Resident's room or housekeeping room—try to eliminate distractions
Materials	Items that were used in common household chores during the time of the resident's childhood. Examples: Metal dish pan, straw broom, old dustpan, butter churn, silver and polishing rag, shoes, shoe polish and brush, rug beater

Benefits

cognitive: defining, describing, giving examples, distin-guishing, labeling, stating, explaining, estimating, re-lating, attention span

physical: fine motor manipulation, basic fine motor and gross motor movements

emotional: enjoyment, expression of frustrations, happi-ness, worthiness, independence

spiritual: recognition of value of work ethic

social: interaction with objects, concept of self, interaction with others

Activity

- Show the resident the chore related items one at a time.
- Encourage the resident to touch and use the items. Dis-cuss how the items were used and how often chores were done.
- Ask what other chores were part of the resident's child-hood.

Conversation Starters

- Do you remember doing chores when you were young?
- What chores were you expected to do?
- When did you do your chores?
- What happened if you did not do your chores?
- What chores did you expect your children to do?

Childhood Pets

Group Size	One on one
Time	10 minutes
Environment	Any quiet place
Materials	Photos of resident's childhood pets
	Photos of pets from magazines
	Toy stuffed animals
	Toy animals from farm sets
	Photos of staff pets

Benefits

emotional: enjoyment, concern (if his/her pet is still alive and with someone else), love, sense of caring for pet

cognitive: describing, identifying, listing, stating, naming, giving examples

spiritual: recognition of the cycles of life

physical: fine motor manipulation

social: interaction with other

Activity

Show resident photos or toy animals. Encourage resident to feel or hold items. Discuss pets that the resident or his/her family had during his/her childhood.

Conversation Starters

- Did you have pets when you were young?
- Did you live in the city or country?
- What were the names of your pets?
- What was your favorite pet?
- Who was responsible for feeding and/or cleaning up after your pet?
- What did you learn from having a pet?

Family Stories

Group Size	One on one
Time	10 to 20 minutes
Environment	Quiet, comfortable area with no distractions
Materials	None necessary—may use tape recorder

Benefits

cognitive: describing, reproducing, explaining, giving examples, relating, composing, creating, sequencing, using language

emotional: satisfaction, enjoyment, excitement, contentment, joy, happiness

spiritual: review family values, sense of "oneness" with family

social: concept of self

Activity

- Every family has "family stories." Tales that have a great deal of meaning to the family. Often these stories are retold at many family gatherings. The stories often involve siblings or extended family.
- Prepare for the activity by asking the family to write or tape some of their stories.
- Start by telling a short story from your family, then ask the resident to tell you one of his/her family stories. If s/he is not able to tell you a story, you can read one of the written stories or play a tape made by a family member.
- If s/he is able to remember stories, make tapes of the telling. Family members will treasure these stories told by the resident.

Conversation Starters

- Can you tell me a story about your family that is told every Christmas? July 4th? etc.
- Who was the favorite family story teller?
- Did you and your brothers or sisters ever do anything that your mother never knew about?

- Do you remember stories your grandparents used to tell? Aunts and uncles?

Family Favorites

Group Size	One on one
Time	10 to 20 minutes
Environment	Quiet, comfortable, appropriate place, i.e. if discussing favorite foods, a kitchen would be appropriate
Materials	Props to use as reminders such as: Photos of places Scents of holidays or seasons Fresh baked bread

Benefits

cognitive: describing, listing, stating, giving examples, relating

emotional: enjoyment, satisfaction, inability to cope, grief (loss of ability), loneliness, desertion, pride, feeling of belonging

spiritual: emphasis on family values

social: interaction with others

Activity

- Prepare by asking family members about favorite family outings, foods, activities, beliefs, etc.
- Share one of your family favorites then ask the resident to tell you about his/her family favorites. Some favorites might include: vacation spots, chores, house or car, holiday, foods.
- If possible, have some props to stimulate memories.
- For those who are unresponsive—relate your family favorites or talk about those supplied by family.

Conversation Starters

- Did your family have reunions? What were they like?
- Did your family spend vacations at relatives? At the beach? Camping?
- Does your family have a special treasured possessions such as a family Bible?
- What foods do you associate with your family?

Photo Poster

Group Size	One on one
Time	20 to 30 minutes
Environment	Quiet room with a large table and comfortable chairs
Materials	Poster board
	Photos of individual's significant life events

Benefits

physical: fine motor manipulation, reaching, possibly crossing mid-line

cognitive: concentrating, selecting, deciding, describing, identifying, labeling, reproducing, giving examples

emotional: satisfaction of reviewing past events, happiness, joy, pride, caring

social: interacting with objects, interacting with others, concept of self

Activity

- Gather pictures and help individual paste pictures of significant life events on poster board. Encourage the individual to talk about his/her history; i.e., childhood, adolescence, wedding, first baby, etc.
- This activity could be used as a family activity. Helpful in cases where the elderly person is no longer able to communicate.
- Pictures from magazines that represent the life events could be used if photos are not available.

Conversation Starters

- Do you have a favorite photo?
- Do you remember your first camera?
- Can you tell me about the people in this picture?
- What would you like to do with this poster? Is there anyone you would like to share it with?

Remembering Different Foods

Group Size	One on one
Time	10 minutes
Environment	Quiet place with a table on which to place pictures or food items
Materials	Pictures of food items cut from magazines and pasted on cardboard Two or three of the individual's favorite food items

Benefits

cognitive: defining, describing, identifying, estimating, selecting

emotional: joy, pleasure from thinking of enjoyable times eating certain foods

social: interacting with others

Activity

Show one picture or food item at a time. Ask the individual to identify the item. Let him/her feel, smell, or taste the food item. Encourage the individual to talk about the food.

Conversation Starters

- What is your favorite food?
- When was the last time you ate your favorite food?
- Show banana—Have you ever had a banana split? Where did you eat banana splits?
- Show strawberry—Do you like strawberry shortcake? When did you eat strawberry shortcake? What occasions?
- Show crackerjack package—Where did you eat cracker jacks? Did you find the prize in the package? Do you remember what the prize was?
- Show potato—What kind of potato do you like best? Did you ever make a face with a potato? What other games did you play with a potato?

Note: Make sure that any food you serve the resident is allowed by his/her physician's current orders regarding food, calorie intake, and consistency. Record all food eaten if that is appropriate.

Childhood Games

Group Size	One on one
Time	10 to 20 minutes
Environment	Resident's room or activity room with table
Materials	Pictures of lay-out of game structure, i.e., lines on floor, hopscotch, shuffle board, 4 square, tic-tac-toe, checkers

Benefits

cognitive: describing, identifying, labeling, giving examples, distinguishing

emotional: enjoyment, satisfaction of remembering success at certain games, enthusiasm, pride

social: interacting with others

Activity

- Introduce activity by asking person, "What games did you play as a child that required you or some object to stay within a pattern of lines?"
- One at a time, show the person a drawing of a game and have him/her guess the name. If s/he can't guess, tell him/her what it is and talk about the object of the game.
- Examples of games: German hopscotch, American hopscotch, shuffle board, 4 square, tic-tac-toe, checkers.

Conversation Starters

- What was your favorite game as a child?
- Who did you play with?
- What did you like about this game?
- What game pieces did you make? How?

Video Contact

Group Size	One on one
Time	15 to 20 minutes
Environment	Quiet area with comfortable chair and video player
Materials	Video of friends or family members: reading a favorite publication telling a familiar story making reassuring comments (Coach the family or friend to use a calm voice and to smile)

Benefits

cognitive: recognizing, concentrating, describing, identifying, reproducing

emotional: comfort at seeing familiar faces, love, happiness

social: reacting to others, interacting with others

Activity

- Play the video for the resident then talk about the topic of the video.
- Often individuals with dementia are unable to distinguish videos from reality. They may think that the person on the video is present in the room. Someone should stay with the resident to stop the video if the resident becomes agitated.

Conversation Starters

- Tell me about that person in the video.
- Do you remember that story (joke, etc.) from the video?

Chapter 6

Occupations and Hobbies

The activities in this chapter focus on occupations and hobbies. Many of the individuals you work with are women who may have never worked away from home. They may not consider that they had a "job." But we all know that making a home comfortable is a valuable, demanding occupation. Housecleaning, laundry, sewing, gardening, all are important activities and for many families were vital in order for the family to function.

Work environments may have been quite different when (and if) the individual was employed. Hours worked, wages and salaries, machinery, procedures, and management styles are much different today. The people you work with have experienced significant changes in their lives and especially in their work lives. It is important to validate the importance of the work they did.

Later life hobbies may have been necessities when they were first started. Gardening, knitting and crocheting, and woodworking may have been necessary to stretch the budget. If the hobby continued over the years it must have given satisfaction and enjoyment as well as providing tangible monetary or other returns. If so, activities that highlight those hobbies can be doubly important!

Individuals with dementia often have trouble with sequencing. That means that any activity that involves following a series of steps will be difficult and may cause agitation. That person may no longer be able to participate in hobbies such as crocheting or cooking that involve following a series of instructions or a recipe, However, s/he may enjoy doing something that involves only one or two steps. S/he may crochet just one long chain or help you make Jell-O. Remember to demonstrate and to give one instruction at a time.

Work Environments

Group Size	One on one
Time	10 to 15 minutes
Environment	Room or area that reflects previous vocations
Materials	Items appropriate to occupation and to type of room in which activity is taking place

Benefits

cognitive: pointing out, describing, distinguishing, labeling, explaining, giving examples, discovering

physical: encourages previously learned patterns of movement

emotional: satisfaction, enjoyment, peacefulness, pride

spiritual: recognition of work ethic

social: interacting with objects, concept of self

Activity

- Take the resident to a room that reflects his/her previous occupation or interest. For instance: kitchen for cook, workshop for manual laborer or hobbyist, office for white collar worker, craft or sewing room for seamstress, library or classroom for teacher
- Allow the resident to handle things in the room, and encourage him/her to look around. Ask what is missing from the room set up.
- Encourage him/her to explain the equipment or to tell how things have changed.
- If possible, ask the person to do a simple task using the area.

Conversation Starters

- Does anything in this room remind you of your work days?
- What is missing that you would normally see when working?
- What equipment did you use in your work?
- What hours did you work?
- How many days a week did you work?

- Do you remember how much you were paid?
- Be aware that many things we use today did not exist when the residents worked. If your office, kitchen, workshop, etc. is very modern, you might import some older equipment.
- Housekeeping rooms with brooms, clothes, mops, etc., where residents can sweep, fold, dust, etc. are helpful for restless residents or those who need to feel useful.

Note: There are very clear federal guidelines against residents working to maintain their living area. If cleaning activity is considered to be therapeutic and therefore done frequently, have this work written up as a care plan objective.

Tools of the Trade

Group Size	One on one
Time	10 to 20 minutes
Environment	Quiet room
Materials	Gender appropriate aprons. Equipment appropriate to occupation or hobby.
	Homemaker—dish cloth, scrubber, measuring spoons, napkin, napkin ring, etc.
	Woodworker—wood, sandpaper, hammer, screw driver, nails and screws, etc.

Benefits

physical: fine motor manipulation, dexterity, tactile stimulation

cognitive: describing, identifying, explaining, giving examples, concentrating

emotional: enjoyment, curiosity

social: interacting with objects, interacting with others, concept of self

Activity

- Help resident to put apron on.
- Show him/her the pockets and allow him/her to explore.
- Encourage the resident to use the equipment.
- Talk about the use of each item.
- Ask if s/he used other similar items.

Conversation Starters

- When did you first begin this occupation or hobby?
- What did you like most about this way of life?
- What would you do differently if you could?
- Who did you teach to do this?
- If the resident is unable to converse—tell the things you know about this occupation or hobby or tell about one of your interests that is similar.

Getting Organized

Group Size	One on one
Time	10 to 15 minutes
Environment	Quiet area with table and chairs
Materials	Small collections of work related items such as: nuts and bolts, washers, and screws
	Kitchen utensils
	Buttons, snaps, and hooks
	Thread or yarn
	Envelopes and other paper such as coupons, paper clips, brads, pens, pencils, hole reinforcers, rubber bands

Benefits

cognitive: distinguishing, identifying, matching, selecting, generalizing, concentrating
physical: fine motor manipulation, dexterity
emotional: satisfaction of doing task, self-confidence
social: interacting with objects

Activity

Scatter collection on the table and ask the resident to sort according to size, color, shape, use, etc. Encourage the resident to talk about the items as s/he sorts.

Conversation Starters

- Do you consider yourself an organized person?
- How did you organize your kitchen (workshop, office, desk, etc.) so you could find things?
- Did you ever have trouble with other people rearranging your space?
- What tools or materials were most important in your work?

Matching Environment to Tools

Group Size	One on one
Time	10 to 20 minutes
Environment	Comfortable room with chairs and a table on which to place objects.
Materials	Pictures of familiar objects or environments associated with the individual's jobs
	Tools associated with various jobs (e.g., slide rule for engineers)

Benefits

cognitive: describing, identifying, matching, selecting, explaining

emotional: expression of feelings of satisfaction, joy of remembering accomplishments, sadness from inability to work any longer

social: interacting with objects, interacting with others, concept of self

physical: fine motor manipulation

Activity

- Give an item to the individual. Find pictures that complement the object and talk to the individual about how the object is used in the work environment.
- The more alert person may be able to tell how the item is used on the job or even tell a story that relates to the object.

Conversation Starters

- What was your occupation?
- Tell me what items you used in your work.
- Did you work alone or with others? Can you tell me about the people you worked with?
- What clothes did you wear to work?
- What hours did you work?

Looking Good

Group Size	One on one
Time	10 to 15 minutes
Environment	Quiet area with table for supplies and comfortable chair for the resident
Materials	Grooming tools
	Women: comb, brush, lotion, liquid makeup, powder, lipstick, cologne, nail file, fingernail polish, herbal facial materials
	Men: comb, electric razor, after-shave, nail file, cologne

Benefits

physical: fine motor manipulation, gross motor movement of arms, stimulating senses

cognitive: describing, selecting, sequencing, following directions

emotional: feeling of satisfaction from looking good, feeling good about someone spending special time

social: concept of self, attention seeking

Activity

- Arrange grooming tools on table, seat the resident and inquire about comfort. Start grooming session with massage (either facial or neck muscles) for relaxation.
- *For women:* Do as much as the person will allow. Encourage her to do as much as she can for herself. Comb or brush the individual's hair. Give her a facial and manicure. Apply makeup and lipstick. Apply cologne or perfume sparingly.
- *For men:* Do as much as the person will allow. Encourage him to do as much as he can for himself. Comb hair, apply hair dressing if he normally uses it. Shave, use after-shave. Give manicure. Apply cologne sparingly.
- Reinforce with compliments about the person's appearance.

**Conversation
Starters**

- What advice did your mother give you about taking care of your hair?
- What services did you use when you went to the beauty shop (barber shop)?
- What color was your hair when you were a child?
- What color hair did the rest of your family have?

Note: Always follow good infection control techniques with all supplies.

Nuts and Bolts

Group Size	One on one
Time	15 to 20 minutes
Environment	Table for materials, comfortable upright chair for the resident
Materials	Various fasteners from a typical workshop: Large screws and nails Nuts and bolts Molly bolts Several plastic containers

Benefits

emotional: enjoyment, feelings of satisfaction in completing a task

cognitive: concentrating, matching skills, visually discriminating, identifying, matching, selecting, explaining

physical: fine motor manipulation, hand-eye coordination

social: interacting with objects

Activity

- Present the resident with a container of mixed fasteners and ask him/her to sort them by size, type, or function. Provide containers for each category. The container could have a picture of the type of fastener on the side.
- This activity may require close supervision to prevent swallowing of the fasteners.

Conversation Starters

- What kind of home workshop did you have?
- Do you consider yourself a "handyman"?
- Tell me how you would use each of these fasteners.

Note: Nails may be considered to be "Sharps" (like needles and scalpels) and may need to be treated with the same precautions. Check with your nursing director before using nails.

Chapter 7

Sports

Sports are a wonderful outlet for many people. The individual may have been actively engaged in sports such as golf, bowling, softball, etc. or have been a spectator and avid fan of a sport. Use that interest any way you can! Help the individual follow his or her favorite team. Banners, tee shirts, and caps with the team logo cue others in to the interest and give even strangers topics of interest to share. Enthusiasm is part of our sports heritage. Use it to your advantage.

Sport Interests

Group Size	One on one
Time	10 to 20 minutes
Environment	Comfortable area with minimal distractions
Materials	Equipment associated with the resident's sports interest: Golf club, fishing rod, baseball, football, tennis racket, boxing gloves

Benefits

cognitive: defining, identifying, reproducing, explaining
physical: fine motor manipulation, gross motor movement
emotional: enjoyment, competitive feelings, expressing frustrations, self-confidence
social: interacting with objects, interacting with others

Activity

Show resident the equipment. Encourage the resident to touch and demonstrate equipment. If resident does not respond, talk about your attempts to use this equipment.

Conversation Starters

- Is this equipment similar to the equipment you used? How is it different?
- Why do you enjoy this particular sport?
- Is there anyone with whom you shared this sport?
- Are you a spectator or active sports person?
- Tell me about some of your adventures in this sport. (Such as attending the World Series, winning a title, bagging a big animal, etc.)

Sports "Grab Bag"

Group Size	One on one
Time	10 to 20 minutes
Environment	An area that has a small table to place the grab bag and items in the bag.
Materials	Three or four items relating to the individual's hobby such as: golf tee, bicycle pant clips, pair of dice, knitting needles, rug hooker, referee's whistle, jacks, thimble, stone for hop scotch, roller skate key, etc.

Benefits

physical: fine motor manipulation

cognitive: problem solving, recalling memories, object identifying

emotional: feelings of joy, excitement

social: interacting with objects, reacting to objects, interacting with others

Activity

- Take out one item at a time. Tell the individual what the item is. Let him/her touch and feel the item. Talk about how the item is used in the particular leisure activity.
- For the individual who is more alert, ask him/her to reach into the bag and feel one item. Can s/he guess what it is? If so, ask him/her to take it out and tell a story using that item as a focus.

Conversation Starters

- What did you do during your playtime as a child? As an adolescent? As an adult?
- Did you ride a bicycle? Where did you ride?
- Did you play card or board games? What is your favorite game?
- Did you make crafts (knitting, crocheting, weaving, sewing)? Tell me about the things you made. What did you do with them?

- Did you roller skate? Where? Ice skate? Where and with whom?

Fanning Football

Group Size	Small group
Time	15 to 20 minutes
Environment	Activity room with lots of space
Materials	Ping-Pong ball, table, newspaper

Benefits

physical: upper body range of motion, strength, eye-hand coordination

cognitive: concentrating, planning strategies, following directions

emotional: joy of accomplishment, competition, excitement, pride

social: interacting with others

Activity

- Two teams line up on opposite sides of the table. Each person uses a folded newspaper to fan the Ping-Pong ball over the opposite side of the table. You can name the teams and keep score.
- Two players can also play this game.

Conversation Starters

- What team games have you played? Did you enjoy going to football, baseball or basketball games?
- Do you remember any cheers from school games?
- What do you like best about this game?

Basketball

Group Size	One on one or small group
Time	10 to 15 minutes
Environment	Large space with no distractions
Materials	Big beach ball or large nerf ball and a large waste basket

Benefits

physical: eye-hand coordination, upper body strength, upper body range of motion

cognitive: concentrating, judging distance, changing performance based on success or failure of last throw

emotional: enjoyment, excitement, feeling of competence

social: interacting with objects, interacting with others

Activity

- Demonstrate throwing the ball into the basket. Give the resident a ball and ask if s/he can make a basket. Start with the basket close to the person. After two or three successful hits, move the basket further away. Change levels by holding the basket in the air or putting it on a chair or table.
- Do not push the person to perform. Allow him/her to perform at his/her own level. Praise all efforts!

Conversation Starters

- Did you ever play basketball?
- What did you wear when you played?
- Did your school have a basketball team? Can you tell me about it?

Bowling

Group Size	One on one or small group
Time	15 to 20 minutes
Environment	Long, narrow space on a bare floor
Materials	Masking tape, large paper cups, large nerf ball

Benefits

physical: eye-hand coordination, upper body range of motion

cognitive: concentrating, estimating, motor planning

emotional: expression of emotions

social: interacting with others, interacting with objects

Activity

- Set up cups (upside down) in the following manner.

- Tape a line about ten feet from the pins. Position the resident on the taped line. The person may stand or sit. Give the person the ball and tell him/her to roll the ball down the floor and see if s/he can knock the pins down. Give him/her two attempts just as in the game of bowling.
- Do not push the person with dementia. Allow him/her to do what s/he can and praise all efforts.

Conversation Starters

- Have you ever bowled before?
- Have you watched others bowl?
- Can you tell me a funny story about bowling?

Target Bean Bag

Group Size	Small group
Time	10 to 15 minutes
Environment	Floor space large enough to fit three concentric circles (e.g. bull's eye) drawn on the floor (1 foot, 1 1/2 foot, and 2 foot)
Materials	Bean bags
	Bean bags may be made with different textured fabrics for more tactile stimulation. They may be made with either beans or macaroni (lighter weight).

Benefits

physical: eye-hand coordination and upper body range of motion

cognitive: concentrating, motor planning, estimating

emotional: satisfaction at doing something successfully, excitement, pride

social: interacting with others, interacting with objects

Activity

- Demonstrate throwing the beanbag into the circles.
- Players sit outside the largest circle and throw three beanbags each. Each person scores 20 points for landing the bag in the outer rim, 50 for the middle, and 100 for the bull's eye.
- For those individuals who are very impaired:
  - Eliminate scoring
  - Use only one circle
  - Do not push
  - Praise all efforts

Conversation Starters

- What does the bean bag feel like?
- What other games involve throwing?

Box Hockey

Group Size	One on one or small group
Time	15 to 20 minutes
Environment	Playing area of 10 x 5 feet with no rug
Materials	Plastic hockey stick
	Nerf hockey puck or ball
	Playing area boundaries
	Wood pieces 4 inches high or improvise with other materials—use 12 inch opening at each end for goal

Benefits

physical: eye-hand coordination, arm and hand strength, and upper body range of motion

cognitive: concentrating, estimating, visually discriminating, following directions

emotional: challenge, feeling of success, joy, excitement, enthusiasm

social: interacting with others, interacting with objects, reacting to objects

Activity

- This activity could be played with one, two, or several residents.
- For one person; set up one goal and let him/her try to hit the puck through the goal.
- For two or more; set up the hockey field with goals at each end. Place the players on each side of the field across from each other. Those on one side are assigned one goal and the others take the goal at the other end of the field. Each player has a hockey stick. Throw the puck in and let the teams try to get the puck in their goal.
- Players who are cognitively impaired may not be able to handle the competitive play. Encourage them to hit the puck with the stick and praise their efforts.

Conversation Starters

- Have you ever played a team game? Tell me about it.
- Have you ever seen a hockey game? What did you like about it?

Chapter 8

Spiritual Pursuit

Spiritual interests are strong in our older generation. It doesn't seem to matter whether the individual has been a part of organized religion; all have a belief system of one sort or another. Over the years they have developed a set of values that have strongly influenced their lives.

One of the tasks of old age is to review our values and our actions to determine if we have met our potential. Have our lives made a difference in this world? To our community? To our families?

The activities in this section will help the individual deal with this issue. Because spiritual issues are a strong influence in an individual's life, they are remembered with meaning after many other functions are gone. Some of these activities may evoke emotions that have not surfaced often or at all. Be prepared to offer support without being judgmental.

Components of Spirituality
by Chuck and Priscilla Sommers

love	hope
praise	embracing
adoration	humbleness
prayer	being present
befriending	faith
compassion	charity
caring	joy
serving	patience
reaching toward another	kindness
"journeying with" (companioning)	goodness
selflessness	faithfulness
gentleness	self-control
forgiving	integration
wholeness	

Values Banner

Group Size	One on one
Time	10 to 20 minutes
Environment	Work table in quiet area
Materials	1/2 yard plain cloth with hem on one end
	2 feet of dowel rod
	Felt, fake fur, beads
	Fabric glue
	Scissors, ruler

Benefits

cognitive: creating, concentrating, describing, identifying, giving examples

physical: fine motor manipulation, hand-eye coordination

emotional: enjoyment, satisfaction

spiritual: review of life values and accomplishments

social: concept of self, interacting with others, interacting with objects

Activity

- Before activity determine some of resident's values through interviews with the resident, family and friends. Nursing staff might also be able to contribute insight.
- Arrange materials on work table. While talking about those things that have been important to the resident, select symbols of those concepts. Assist the resident in cutting out symbols and gluing them to the banner. Run dowel rod through top of banner and hang for display.

Conversation Starters

- What people are most important to you? Ideas? Possessions?
- If you won $1,000 unexpectedly, what would you do with it?
- What would you want people to say about you when you die?

Spiritual Moments

Group Size	One on one
Time	15 to 20 minutes
Environment	Quiet area—may wish to have religious symbols or flowers in room
Materials	Bible or pertinent religious book
	Personal religious items (e.g. rosary)
	Taped message from pastor or other inspirational message
	Tape of inspirational music
	Tape from resident's Sunday school class or prayer group

Benefits

emotional: enjoyment, fulfillment, love, hopefulness, relief, peacefulness

spiritual: reflection on personal meaning of religion, reaffirmation of values, reflection on meaning of life

cognitive: identifying, recognizing names, describing

social: concept of self, interaction with others

Activity

- Play tape of message or music for resident.
- If possible remain with resident, be available to hold hands or otherwise show support.
- Discuss thoughts inspired by the tape.

Conversation Starters

- What religious event has meant the most to you? Why?
- Do you have a favorite hymn? Would you like to sing it?
- Did you take part in the services at your church? In the Women's (or Men's) groups?
- Do you remember church socials?
- Did you belong to your church youth group? What was important about that group?

Heavenly Food

Group Size	One on one
Time	10 to 15 minutes
Environment	Comfortable dining area with minimal distractions.
Materials	Food normally associated with a religious event such as: Easter eggs, candy cane, wedding cake, hot-cross buns, matzo

Benefits

cognitive: describing, distinguishing, identifying, explaining, relating, classifying

physical: sense of taste, fine motor manipulation, jaw movements

emotional: enjoyment, contentment

spiritual: reminder of spiritual milestones

social: reacting to objects, interacting with others

Activity

- Show food to resident. Help the resident to feel, smell, and taste. Encourage the resident to tell memories brought to mind by the food.
- The resident who is less responsive might still enjoy the smell and taste of the food. Talk about the traditions and the religious significance of the food.

Conversation Starters

- What event do you associate with this food?
- Did you take part in preparing holiday food in your home? Church? Tell me how those foods were prepared.
- What other foods do you associate with holidays or religious events?

Note: Make sure that any food you serve the resident is allowed by his/her physician's current orders regarding food, calorie intake, and consistency. Report all food eaten if that is appropriate.

Books of Faith

Group Size	One on one
Time	10 to 15 minutes
Environment	Quiet, comfortable place—perhaps in the chapel
Materials	Books of the resident's faith
	Bible or old book of children's bible stories
	Prayer book
	"Guideposts" or other publications
	Book of daily meditation

Benefits

cognitive: recognizing words, discriminating visually, identifying, naming, describing, giving examples

emotional: enjoyment, satisfaction, love, relief, peacefulness

spiritual: renewed feelings of faith

social: interacting with objects, interacting with others

Activity

- Select one or two books the resident enjoys. (Ask family or friends for suggestions.) Show one book to the resident at a time. Encourage the resident to read the book out loud if s/he is able. Otherwise, read favorite passages or stories to the resident.
- For the less responsive; use old children's picture books that might be familiar to him/her. Talk about the stories represented by the photos.
- This is a good activity for the resident's friends from church.

Conversation Starters

- Do you have a favorite Bible story? Why do you like that story?
- Can you name the books of the Bible?
- Have you ever read the Bible through?
- Which stories do you think might help a child today? A young parent? An old person?

61

Heroes

Group Size	One on one or small group
Time	10 to 15 minutes
Environment	Quiet, comfortable place
Materials	Photos of heroes from the 30's, 40's, and 50's: Teddy Roosevelt, Franklin Roosevelt, Charles Lindbergh, Admiral Bird, Amelia Earhart, Generals Patton and Eisenhower, Billy Graham, Frank Sinatra, Betty Grabel
	Tapes of radio programs featuring a hero

Benefits

cognitive: matching name/face, defining, describing, distinguishing, selecting, giving examples, comparing

emotional: enjoyment, sense of pride, importance, confidence

spiritual: clarification of personal and societal values

social: interacting with others, reacting to objects

Activity

- Come equipped with photos of heroes or tapes of old radio presentations of heroes. Ask the resident who his/her personal hero was. Talk about your collection one at a time. Listen to the tape or look at the photos. Encourage the resident to talk about the heroes. S/he might like to bring mementos of his/her personal heroes.
- For the non-responsive—talk about people you admire. Tell the resident what you most admire about him/her.

Conversation Starters

- Who is your favorite hero?
- Do you consider someone in your family a hero? Why?
- What do you admire most about your hero?
- Have you ever been a hero? What was the reaction of your friends and family?
- Who did you most admire when you were young? How did that person influence your life?

This Is Who I Am

Group Size	One on one or small group
Time	15 to 20 minutes
Environment	Quiet area with table and chairs
Materials	Old magazines with photos
	Scissors
	Posterboard and glue

Benefits
physical: hand-eye coordination, hand and upper body range of motion

cognitive: distinguishing, identifying, labeling, reproducing, stating, giving examples, generalizing, compiling

emotional: pleasure of accomplishment, love, happiness, sadness, dealing with loneliness, importance, peacefulness, pride

spiritual: recognition of value as a person

social: concept of self, interacting with objects, interacting with others

Activity
- Help the resident look through the magazines and select photos of things s/he likes. Then help him/her to cut those photos out and glue to poster board which is cut to size of the pictures. These may be laminated for durability.
- These picture cards can be used to talk about the person's likes and may be displayed in the room for others to use as conversation clues.

Conversation Starters
- For each picture selected ask "What do you like about this item or place?"

Chapter 9

Places Lived and Visited

The individual who has lost his or her ability to function independently has experienced devastating losses. Often that includes his or her home and certainly the ability to travel. One's home is the heart of the family. Each home is unique, reflecting the people who live there. A person who can't remember where s/he left his/her glasses may, and frequently will, recite every detail of his/her childhood bedroom.

Not all folks were travelers, but those who had the opportunity and the inclination usually enjoyed the experience. From the very successful trips to the disasters, they are all remembered with fondness.

This group of activities will help the individual to enjoy memories of his or her home, community, and important places s/he has visited.

Town, People, and Places

Group Size	One on one
Time	10 to 20 minutes
Environment	Quiet area with comfortable chairs
Materials	Photos of old buildings and well-known places
	Video tapes of town and people
	Audio tapes of familiar town sounds
	Well-known products of town
	Samples of food popular in town

Benefits

cognitive: describing, distinguishing, identifying, giving examples

emotional: enjoyment, expressing sadness and loss

spiritual: recognition of continuity in life

social: reacting to objects, interacting with others, concept of self

Activity

- Show the resident photos of well-known places, buildings, or people (from his/her younger years if s/he has dementia). Ask the resident if s/he recognizes any of the photos. If so, ask him/her to tell you about them.
- Show the resident video tapes of the town and people (perhaps some members of his/her family). Ask the resident to respond to the video.
- Play audio tapes of familiar sounds. Follow up on any response from the resident.
- Show the resident products or food and ask if s/he can identify them. Allow him/her to handle the items.

Conversation Starters

- What did you like best about this town?
- What streets did you use most often?
- Tell me about the grade school (or high school) you attended. Is it still there?
- Did your brothers and sisters attend the same schools? Your children? Grandchildren?

- What did you do in your free time? In the summer? Winter?

Memories of Home

<table>
<tr><td>Group Size</td><td>One on one</td></tr>
<tr><td>Time</td><td>15 to 20 minutes</td></tr>
<tr><td>Environment</td><td>Comfortable, quiet, home-like room</td></tr>
<tr><td>Materials</td><td>Items from the resident's home or room.
For instance: figurines, doilies, pillows, afghans, books, old clock, or radio</td></tr>
</table>

Benefits

cognitive: describing, distinguishing, identifying, stating, explaining, giving examples, calculating, contrasting

emotional: warm feelings of home, enjoyment, satisfaction, expression of sadness or loneliness

physical: fine motor manipulation

social: interacting with objects, concept of self, interacting with others

Activity

- Using one object at a time, comment on the object, ask what it was used for in the home. Encourage the resident to handle the object. Ask if there are any special stories about the object.
- For the resident who is less responsive: talk about the object. Describe it in detail, speculate about what roles it may have played in the home. Relate any stories you have heard from family or friends about the resident's home.

Conversation Starters

- Can you describe your home to me? What was your favorite room in your house? Why?
- Did you buy or rent your home?
- Who were your neighbors?
- How long did you live in your house? Or in each house?
- What was different about the neighborhood when you first lived there?

Music of Other Places

<table>
<tr><td>Group Size</td><td>One on one or small group</td></tr>
<tr><td>Time</td><td>10 to 30 minutes</td></tr>
<tr><td>Environment</td><td>Table big enough to place musical instruments</td></tr>
<tr><td>Materials</td><td>Bongo drums, maracas, mouth harp, tambourines, cassette tapes, tape player</td></tr>
</table>

Benefits

cognitive: describing, distinguishing, matching, explaining, summarizing

emotional: laughter, joy, peacefulness

social: interacting with objects, interacting with others

Activity

- Take one instrument at a time and demonstrate rhythmical sound.
- Discuss where the instrument originated.
- Play a tape of music which focuses on this instrument.
- Ask the person where this music originated.

Conversation Starters

- What type of dance is done to this music?
- Where in the United States have you visited? The world?
- What places have you lived?
- What type of music was popular in the places you have lived or visited?

Travel Log

Group Size	Small group
Time	20 to 30 minutes
Environment	Comfortable room with minimum distractions
Materials	Slides, videos, music

Benefits

cognitive: describing, identifying, listing, explaining, giving examples

emotional: pleasant memories, curiosity, peacefulness, enthusiasm, carefreeness

social: reaction to others

Activity

- Ask a volunteer to come in and share with the residents a trip s/he took, using slides, music, and narrative.
- Or present a video travel log.

Conversation Starters

- What do you know about this place?
- What places have you visited?
- Who went with you on trips?
- Did you take photos? Tell me about your camera.

Dances from Foreign Places

Group Size	One on one or small group
Time	15 to 20 minutes
Environment	Space enough for a small group to dance
Materials	Records, tapes of dances from foreign countries

Benefits

physical: large muscle, cardiovascular exercise
cognitive: motor planning, sequencing, describing, identifying, giving examples, reproducing
emotional: enjoyment, satisfaction, pride, enthusiasm
social: interacting with others

Activity

- Put records/tapes on and let a volunteer group perform some ethnic dance. Then ask residents in which country this particular dance originated. Waltz, polka, cha-cha, square dance, are examples.
- If residents are able, let them take part in the dancing.

Conversation Starters

- Did you dance when you were younger?
- What types of dances did you do?
- Have you ever seen a group perform dances from another country?
- What did you like best about this dance?

Chapter 10

Artistic Interests

The activities in this section provide an opportunity for creative expression. Most of us have a capacity for artistic expression that has gone untapped. Many older folks were raised in an era when "artsy stuff" may have been considered "a waste of time." However, creating an artistic piece can give one a sense of satisfaction and increase one's self-esteem.

In addition to being creative, some of these activities also produce "useful" items. All efforts should be praised for their artistic value and uses for the creation should be discussed.

During artistic activities, you might consider playing soft, flowing music that will help form images in the mind and create a relaxing background for the artistic endeavor.

Creative Beauty

Group Size	Small group
Time	30 to 45 minutes
Environment	Large table area for each resident
Materials	Pan for water
	Sponge
	Finger paint or poster paint
	Pudding
	Glazed paper
	News print or tissue paper

Benefits

physical: hand-eye coordination, upper body range of motion

cognitive: following directions, creating, monitoring one's work and adjusting actions to achieve desired outcome

emotional: satisfaction, enjoyment

social: interacting with objects, interacting with others, reacting to objects

Activity

- This activity is a good way to express feelings or to enjoy the sense of touch. There are no hard and fast rules. Just let yourself create.
- Lay the glazed paper on a hard surface, moisten the paper with a wet sponge, and smooth it to disperse any bubbles. Put dabs of paint or pudding onto the paper with a spoon, then work it over the paper with fingers, palm, or ball of the hand. All of these can be used to execute a design. A pattern will emerge which then can be given more definition, with the fingers or hands. A second color may be added over the first to add expression and beauty to the design.
- When dry, the paper can be used for gift-wrapping, covering boxes, or even as a framed picture.

Conversation Starters

- Have you ever done anything like this before?
- What do you think you will do with this painting?
- What similar activities have you done in the past with your fingers that had the same feeling?

Note: If you use only the primary colors of red, blue, and yellow, you will be less likely to end up with brown or muddied pictures.

Awareness Cards

Group Size	Small group
Time	20 to 30 minutes
Environment	Well lighted area with table and chairs
Materials	Poster board, scissors, magazines

Benefits

physical: eye-hand coordination, fine motor manipulation

cognitive: concentrating, defining, describing, distinguishing, identifying, explaining

emotional: love, joy, peacefulness, sympathy, pride, caring

social: interacting with others, interacting with objects

Activity

- This activity would make a good intergenerational activity. Individuals who are more alert could help those with limited functioning.
- Find thought-provoking pictures of past (such as World War II) or present events and cut out. Paste on poster board of the same size (no smaller than 5 x 6). May be laminated to keep clean.
- The cards can be used to tell stories, elicit memories, or talk about changes in the world.

Conversation Starters

- Focus on the picture selected. Do you remember this event?
- Were you there? If not, where were you when it happened?
- How did you hear about it?
- How do you keep up with current events?

Expression Through Art

Group Size	One on one or small group
Time	15 to 30 minutes
Environment	Quiet area with table and chairs
Materials	Clay or play dough
	Items to make impressions in the clay or to cut the clay
	Paper (newsprint)
	Marker

Benefits

physical: fine motor manipulation, eye-hand coordination

cognitive: concentrating, expressing creativity, changing, manipulating, modifying, producing, showing, constructing

emotional: confidence, self-esteem, sense of identity, contentment

social: interacting with objects, concept of self

Activity

- Ask the individual to make something from the clay that is an expression of his/her personal experiences.
- The resident who is less responsive may enjoy just making shapes (such as snakes) out of the clay.
- Another approach is to give the individual a marker and paper and ask him/her to draw a self portrait or a picture of something s/he likes.

Conversation Starters

- Tell me how this sculpture/drawing reflects your experiences.
- Tell me about this portrait.
- Have you made anything from clay before? What?
- If you could change your self-portrait how would you do it?
- What do you do that is creative?

Sponge Painting

Group Size	One on one or small group
Time	15 to 30 minutes
Environment	Quiet room with table large enough for materials and work space
Materials	Sponges cut into different shapes
	Acrylic paints of different colors
	Thick white paper

Benefits

physical: eye-hand coordination, fine motor manipulation

cognitive: concentrating, creating, modifying, visually discriminating, arranging

emotional: satisfaction with expressing, creating and making useful item, joy, pride

social: interacting with others, interacting with objects

Activity

- Assist the resident to choose a sponge and paint color.
- Dip sponge into paint and press on paper.
- Paper can be used as gift wrap or framed for show.

Conversation Starters

- Did you ever make your own gift wrapping?
- What did you use to wrap your gifts?
- What special things did you use to make it creative?
- What was the most unusual wrapping you ever received?

Remembering Holidays

Group Size	One on one or small group
Time	20 to 30 minutes
Environment	Table with space for cookie cutters and drawing materials
Materials	Cookie cutters with shapes representing different holidays of the year, white paper, markers

Benefits

physical: fine motor manipulation, eye-hand coordination

cognitive: sequencing, describing, identifying symbols, listing, matching, selecting, distinguishing, giving examples

emotional: pride, satisfaction, joy, happiness, enthusiasm

social: interacting with others, interacting with objects

spiritual: associating holidays with religious significance, reawakening sense of values

Activity

- Outline cookie cutter shape with marker. Decorate with other colored markers.
- Ask the resident what holidays are represented by the different shapes, i.e., Valentine's day, Christmas, Easter, Halloween.
- Ask the resident to place cookie cutters in order according to when the holidays occur during the year (only if you know the resident has the ability to sequence).
- Trace cookie cutter shapes on light weight cardboard. Cut out shape and punch a hole (for hanging) near the top of the shape. Have the resident glue uncooked noodles onto the shape. After the glue dries, spray paint the shape and attach a pretty ribbon on which it can hang.

Conversation Starters

- Do you remember times when you baked cookies for special occasions? Where? Who were you with?
- What kinds of cookies did you make? Which were your favorite?

Chapter 11

Drama and Laughter

Humor is an essential characteristic of every human being. It is an over-learned response. From the time we are born, people are trying to make us smile and laugh. For some people humor is a very effective coping devise. Humor relieves tension and aids communication. Our sense of humor stays with us throughout our lives.

We tend to forget that individuals who are low functioning have a sense of humor. They have suffered so many losses that we think they should feel only sadness. Sometimes we react to their attempts at humor negatively—thinking that they are exhibiting signs of confusion or hallucinating. When we recognize the humor in another, we validate their existence as a humorous person. Tension is released, self-esteem is increased, trust is established and communication is enhanced.

Jokes require cognitive abilities. One must understand the punch line. Some individuals who are impaired may have lost that ability. But humor is far more than jokes with punch lines. There are many funny situations and things that will delight the individual. If you are having fun, the chances are that the person you are working with will have fun also!

The Joke's on You

Group Size	One on one
Time	10 minutes
Environment	Quiet area with comfortable seating
Materials	Books of simple jokes
	Large cartoons
	Magazines with funny stories, limericks or jokes

Benefits

cognitive: stimulating sense of humor, distinguishing, comparing, identifying, inferring, identifying "what is wrong with this situation?"

physical: increased circulation (with hearty laughter), relaxation

emotional: enjoyment, happiness

social: reacting to others, interacting with others

Activity

- Humor is very important for individuals who are cognitively impaired. The sense of humor often remains intact long after other faculties are gone.
- Make the resident comfortable. Tell him/her that you have found some jokes s/he might enjoy. Read simple jokes or share cartoons. Be sure to keep the jokes simple. Some residents may not be able to grasp the concept of the joke. However you may find him/her laughing because you are laughing.
- Encourage the resident to tell you a joke or funny story. Remember to LAUGH!

Conversation Starters

- What (or who) makes you laugh?
- Do you have a favorite joke? Cartoon?
- What kind of jokes do you like best? One liners, limericks, shaggy dog stories?
- Do you remember a time when the joke was on you?

Comedy Props

Group Size	One on one
Time	10 to 15 minutes
Environment	Quiet, comfortable place
Materials	Props that are fun to look at or to feel, such as: Windmills, bubbles, koosh balls, false noses, oversized glasses, mechanical trick toys, funny hats

Benefits

cognitive: defining, describing, distinguishing, explaining, generalizing, giving examples, matching names to actions

physical: fine motor manipulation

emotional: enjoyment, laughter, enthusiasm, carefreeness

social: interacting with objects, reacting to objects, interacting with others

Activity

- Have two or three props handy. Show the resident one prop at a time. Encourage the resident to feel and use the item.
- If the resident is unresponsive, help him/her to hold the item. Describe the item and tell a story about it.

Conversation Starters

- What or who makes you laugh?
- What makes a baby laugh?
- Do you remember the Marx brothers? The Three Stooges? Lucy? Charlie Chaplin? Buster Keaton? What did they do that made you laugh?
- Have you ever laughed so hard you cried? Tell me about it.

Action Songs

Group Size	One on one or small group
Time	10 to 15 minutes
Environment	Quiet area
Materials	Recordings of motion songs (optional)

Benefits

physical: stretching, fine motor manipulation, motor coordination

cognitive: concentrating, remembering, sequencing, identifying, reproducing

emotional: enjoyment, peacefulness, enthusiasm, pride, security

social: interacting with others

Activity

- Invite the resident to join you in singing and acting out songs. Use songs that the person may have sung as a child or to his/her children. Lead in the motions as the resident follows or gently guide the person through the song by holding his/her hands and doing the motions.
- Songs: Row, Row, Row Your Boat; I'm a Little Teapot; Itsy Bitsy Spider; Rock-a-Bye Baby.

Conversation Starters

- Do you have a favorite song?
- What part of these songs do you like best?
- What songs made you laugh? What songs made your children laugh?

Leading the Band

Group Size	One on one or small group
Time	10 to 20 minutes
Environment	Comfortable area with record, CD, or tape player
Materials	Record or tape of band or orchestra music
	Baton (could use cardboard tube)
	Scarves, pom-poms, flags, or wooden spoons

Benefits

physical: upper body range of motion

cognitive: concentrating, using rhythm, following directions, sequencing, determining beat, matching

emotional: enjoyment, love, excitement, importance, peacefulness, enthusiasm, pride

social: interacting with objects, reacting to others (rhythm)

Activity

- Play music with a good beat. Demonstrate leading the band with a baton. Give the resident a baton and suggest s/he follow your lead.
- Provide rest periods as needed. Watch for fatigue. Smile!

Conversation Starters

- How does leading a band make you feel?
- Did you ever play in a band? Sung in a chorus?
- Who was your favorite "big band" leader?
- Who was your favorite "big band" singer?

Poems, Limericks, and Stories

Group Size	One on one
Time	15 to 20 minutes
Environment	Comfortable space with minimal distractions
Materials	Limericks, poems and stories that might be familiar to the resident

Benefits

cognitive: concentrating, associating words, recognizing patterns, describing, identifying, reproducing, explaining, giving examples

emotional: enjoyment, laughter, love, satisfaction, happiness, peacefulness, enthusiasm, pride, caring

social: interacting with others

Activity

- Read limericks, poems or stories, leaving out the key words and wait for the resident to fill in those words before proceeding. Example:

    Roses are _____ (color),
    Violets are _____ (color),
    (Desert) _____ is sweet,
    And so is _____ (name).
    OR
    'Twas the night before …

- Many people can recite old familiar poems and stories long after other memories are gone. Give the person plenty of time to find the word, but do not press him/her. Supply the answer before s/he becomes agitated.

Conversation Starters

- Do you have a favorite poem, limerick or story that you can tell me?
- Do you remember memorizing poems in school?

Chapter 12

Cognitive Challenges

As a society we are beginning to recognize the value of physical exercise in keeping the body physically fit. There is also value in keeping cognitively fit. These exercises stimulate cognitive functioning. They exercise the memory, encourage concentration, and reward effective problem solving.

Some of these activities may be frustrating for the adult with dementia. However there may be cognitive abilities remaining that will surface with stimulation. Try one part of an activity at a time. You may have to try several times. Always stop the activity if the individual becomes agitated. Your knowledge of the resident and your judgment skills will guide you, but do not be afraid or hesitant to try. The resident may surprise you!

Jigsaw Puzzle

Group Size	One on one
Time	10 to 20 minutes
Environment	Quiet area with table and chairs
Materials	Cereal box cut up into jagged pieces

Benefits

cognitive: concentrating, defining, describing, distinguishing, identifying, matching, reproducing, predicting, modifying

physical: eye-hand coordination, fine motor manipulation

emotional: sense of satisfaction, achievement, self-confidence, happiness, enthusiasm

social: interacting with objects, interacting with others

Activity

- Spread pieces of the puzzle on a flat table and ask the resident to piece them together. If s/he is having difficulty, do it with him/her.
- After the puzzle is completed, compliment the resident on a job well done.
- Talk about the cereal box, i.e. the brand name, the type of cereal, whether or not s/he ever ate this type, etc.

Conversation Starters

- Have you ever put together a jigsaw puzzle?
- What type of puzzles do you like best?
- What type of cereal did you eat when you were a child?
- What kind of cereal do you like best now?

Note: Keep a variety of "puzzles" around. Have at least one puzzle made up of just 2 pieces, a few with just 3 pieces, etc.

Different Textured Puzzles

Group Size	One on one
Time	10 to 15 minutes
Environment	Quiet area with table and chairs
Materials	Cardboard, burlap, satin, medium weight plastic, velvet, sand paper

Benefits

physical: fine motor manipulation, hand-eye coordination, tactile stimulation

cognitive: concentrating, defining, identifying, recognizing, matching, reproducing, predicting, modifying

emotional: satisfaction, curiosity, hopefulness, self-confidence, excitement, peacefulness, pleasure

social: interacting with objects, interacting with others, reacting to objects

Activity

- For each piece of material, cut out a shape (circle, triangle, heart, other geometrical shape). Each shape is then cut into several pieces. Put all pieces into a box. Encourage the individual to pick out pieces and match them by texture.
- When all pieces have been separated, puzzles can be put together.
- Individuals who are visually impaired particularly enjoy this activity.
- The number of pieces can vary according to the functioning level of the individual.
- Have some of the puzzles made up of just two or three pieces.

Conversation Starters

- What does this fabric (or other material) remind you of?
- Did you sew? What did you make?
- What fabric do you like to wear? Why?
- What else has distinctive textures?

Alphabet Bags

Group Size	One on one
Time	10 to 30 minutes
Environment	Quiet area with comfortable chairs and a table
Materials	Paper bags filled with a variety of objects

Benefits

physical: tactile sense, fine motor manipulation

cognitive: concentrating, defining, describing, distinguishing, identifying, labeling, matching, explaining

emotional: enjoyment, challenge, self-confidence, satisfaction, happiness, enthusiasm, pride

social: interacting with objects

Activity

- Label paper bags with each letter of the alphabet. Fill each bag with one or more items beginning with that letter and have the individual guess the object by feel.
- Examples: apple, bobby pin, cork, dice, earring, fork, golf ball, half dollar, ice cube tray, jar, key, lemon, match, nut, orange, pipe, quill, ruler, spool, thimble, undershirt, vegetable, wishbone, letter X cut from cardboard, yarn, and a zipper.

Conversation Starters

- Tell me what this object makes you think of.
- How did you learn your ABC's?

Buttons

Group Size	One on one
Time	10 to 15 minutes
Environment	Quiet area with table and chairs
Materials	Container for buttons—sets of 5 to 10 in different sizes, colors, textures, or shapes
	Container with several compartments such as egg carton or apple crate separator

Benefits

physical: fine motor manipulation, hand-eye coordination

cognitive: classifying, sorting according to color, size, shape, or texture, following directions, matching, explaining

emotional: feeling of satisfaction from being successful, pride, usefulness

social: interacting with objects, interacting with others

Activity

- Let the resident feel different textures and sizes of buttons. Put three buttons (two the same and one different) in front of him/her and ask him/her to pick out the one that is different than the other two. Ask him/her to pick out three buttons that are the same color or same size or same texture.
- Individuals who are more alert may be able to sort larger numbers of buttons in a variety of ways.

Conversation Starters

- Can you think of any other ways to sort these buttons?
- What do these buttons remind you of?
- Which button do you like best? Why?
- Where (in your house) did you keep your extra buttons?
- What materials are buttons made of?
- What games are played with buttons?

Jars and Lids

Group Size	One on one
Time	10 to 15 minutes
Environment	Quiet area with table and chairs
Materials	Different sizes and shapes of jars, bottles and lids, some plastic and some glass

Benefits

physical: fine motor manipulation, eye-hand coordination

cognitive: size and shape discriminating, observing size relationships, making comparisons, assembling, selecting, matching, distinguishing, identifying, problem solving

emotional: satisfaction of completing a task, independence

social: interacting with others, interacting with objects

Activity

- Ask the individual to:
  - match lids with the jars
  - place jars in order of height
  - place lids in order of size
  - make a pattern on the table using jars and lids
- Activity staff makes pattern and asks individual to copy the pattern using other jars and lids

Conversation Starters

- Which jar has the biggest lid?
- What do you think this jar held?
- What type of item do you think this jar was made for?
- Do you remember using old jars for storing things? What did you store?
- Did you can fruits and vegetables? What did you like to can best?

Money Matters

Group Size	One on one
Time	5 to 10 minutes
Environment	Uncluttered area with a table
Materials	Quarters, nickels, dimes, and pennies

Benefits

physical: fine motor manipulation

cognitive: defining, describing, calculating, identifying, matching, reproducing, converting, giving examples, changing

emotional: pride, happiness

social: interacting with others, interacting with objects

Activity

- For the adult with dementia, allow the individual to handle one coin at a time. Tell him/her the name of each coin. Show him/her the different combinations that total 25 cents.
- Ask the resident who is more alert to name each coin. See if s/he can make a combination that equals 25 cents. See if s/he can come up with three combinations that total 25 cents. Ask him/her to total all the coins, (The resident may need a pencil and paper to do this.)
- It might be helpful to show an example of coin combinations as you work with the individual.

Conversation Starters

- What kinds of things were you able to buy for a quarter? For a dime? For a nickel?
- Do you remember when you first started saving your money? How did you do that?
- Did you use the "postal savings" program at school? How much money did you give for offering at Sunday school or church when you were a child?
- Did you get an allowance? How much?
- What were the first jobs you remember doing for money?

Sequencing Cards

Group Size	One on one
Time	15 to 20 minutes
Environment	Table large enough to spread out cards
Materials	Sets of three 5" x 8" cardboard cards with three scene sequential stories drawn on the cards. *Example: 1)* Woman taking apples out of basket; 2) Woman baking pie; 3) Woman eating pie. *Alternate example*: 1) Mailman putting letter in mailbox; 2) man opening the mailbox; 3) man reading letter inside house.

Benefits

cognitive: sequencing, interpreting pictures, distinguishing, identifying, reproducing, explaining, changing

emotional: self-confidence, frustration, satisfaction, happiness, enthusiasm, pride

social: interacting with others, interacting with objects

Activity

- Ask the resident to put cards in order of how things occur. Talk about memories triggered by stories.
- May use photos cut from magazines instead of drawings.
- For those residents with severe dementia, try using two card sequences.

Conversation Starters

- Can you tell me a story about these pictures?
- Do you like to do this activity? (Baking, sending and receiving letters, etc.)

Matching Colors

Group Size	One on one
Time	15 to 20 minutes
Environment	Quiet space with a table
Materials	Make a wooden base (8" x 14") with five dowels of different lengths and colors fastened to it
	Make colored cardboard discs with holes to fit over dowel. Paint same color as dowels.

Benefits

physical: fine motor manipulation, hand-eye coordination

cognitive: concentrating, sequencing, counting, matching, identifying, describing

emotional: success, frustration, self-confidence, satisfaction, enthusiasm, pride

Activity

- Ask the resident to match the discs with the dowels by color.
- Number the dowels consecutively and have the resident place the appropriate number of discs on each dowel.

Conversation Starters

- What is your favorite color?
- Can you see this color anywhere else in the room?
- What colors do you see around you?

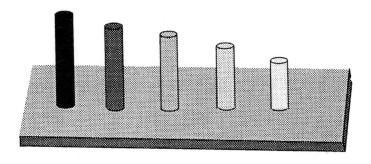

Name Recognition

Group Size	One on one
Time	5 to 10 minutes
Environment	Quiet area with table and chairs
Materials	Paper, marker, felt or plastic letters

Benefits

physical: eye-hand coordination, fine motor manipulation

cognitive: concentrating, distinguishing, identifying, reproducing, selecting, rewriting, compiling

emotional: feeling of success, self-confidence, happiness, pride

social: interacting with others, interacting with objects

Activity

- Print the resident's name in large print on a piece of paper. Provide letters and ask the person to select appropriate letters that spell his/her name.
- Those with very limited functioning may be able to do this with just the letters in their name. Others will be able to select correct letters from the entire alphabet.

Conversation Starters

- Do you have a nickname? What is it?
- What do you like best about your name?
- What other names do you like?

Holidays and Seasons

Group Size	One on one or small group
Time	15 to 20 minutes
Environment	Quiet space with comfortable seating
Materials	Large calendar with seasonal pictures at the top of each month

Benefits

cognitive: describing, distinguishing, identifying, listing, matching, sequencing, giving examples

emotional: love, satisfaction, joy, happiness, expression of sadness or loneliness, peacefulness, enthusiasm, security

social: interacting with others

Activity

- Hold calendar up to show the month of the year you wish to talk about.
- Ask the residents what holiday or special event occurs during the month.
  - January—New Year's Day, M. L. King Day
  - February—Valentine's Day
  - March—St. Patrick's Day
  - April—April Fool's Day, Easter
  - May—May Day, Mother's Day
  - June—Father's Day, Summer Vacation
  - July—Fourth of July
  - August—Back to school
  - September—Labor Day
  - October—Columbus Day
  - November—Veteran's Day, Thanksgiving
  - December—Hanukkah, Christmas
  - Add well-known local events.
- Discuss what kind of weather one could expect during the month. Talk about the changing seasons.

Conversation Starters

- What are the trees doing during this month?
- What flowers would you see?
- What clothes would you wear?

97

Chapter 13

Physical Activities

The remaining activities in this book are activities that are important to the resident who is impaired, but which may not relate specifically to his/her previous experiences.

Physical activities help the individual maintain physical abilities. These activities help promote circulation, encourage range of motion, strength, endurance, coordination and enhance body image. These physical activities are important and should be a regular part of an activity care plan for the person with physical or cognitive limitations.

Physical activities often give opportunities for non-threatening touch. Appropriate touch can convey caring and approval. Holding hands, hugs, an arm around a shoulder, and shaking hands, all are appropriate if the resident does not draw away and indicate that s/he does not want to be touched. For many residents caring touches are rare. This is an opportunity for you to make a real difference in his/her life.

Physical activities can be strenuous, so keep the movements slow and plan frequent rest breaks. Limit the variety in any one activity, demonstrate the activity, and give instructions one at a time (checking for understanding each time). To help reduce fatigue, try not to use the same muscle groups for any two activities. Whenever possible, start with lower body exercises first, then work up to the upper body exercises. This will help reduce the strain on the resident's heart.

Relaxing Movement

Group Size	One on one or small group
Time	15 to 20 minutes
Environment	Enough space to be able to stretch arms and legs in all directions
Materials	Tapes of instrumental music in slow and fast rhythms

Benefits

physical: cardiovascular exercise, upper body range of motion by stretching, breath control

cognitive: following sequences of movement patterns, identifying, naming, giving examples

emotional: provides a way to accept new body boundaries and feeling good about remaining capacity (capability)

social: interacting with others, interacting with objects (rhythm)

Activity

- Put some slow instrumental music on and do some easy stretches and bends with legs, torso, neck, and arms. Breath slowly in and out with the music.
- If the resident is unable to follow, direct movements by holding on to hands and lifting arms together. Gently lift legs and stretch.
- Put on music with a quick beat. Ask the resident to follow your movements. Clap your hands together with the beat, tap knees with hands, tap toes on floor.
- Put waltz music on. Hold hands of the resident and dance the waltz step while s/he feels the rhythm through your movements.

Conversation Starters

- Do you remember doing special dances to this music?
- What kind of dancing did you enjoy the most?

Note: Always start with lower extremity exercises first. This moves blood up from the lower extremities and reduces the degree of stress on the heart.

Balloon Ball

Group Size	One on one or small group
Time	15 to 20 minutes
Environment	Space for a small group to sit in a circle with about a foot of space between each chair
Materials	16 inch balloon

Benefits

physical: upper and lower body range of motion, eye-hand coordination

cognitive: concentrating, recognizing handedness, distinguishing, describing

emotional: pride, satisfaction, happiness, excitement, enthusiasm

social: interacting with objects, reacting to objects, interacting with others

Activity

- Ask the resident to hit the balloon with both hands across the circle. See if s/he can hit with just his/her right hand or just his/her left hand. Now let him/her kick the balloon with his/her feet.
- Residents who are restricted to their beds can also participate one-on-one with a volunteer, family member or activity staff.

Conversation Starters

- What events involve balloons?
- Do you like to blow up balloons? Pop them?
- How long do you think a balloon would stay inflated if no one broke it?
- What places do you often see balloons? (fairs, circuses, florist shops, birthday parties, etc.)

Balloons and Balls

Group Size	One on one
Time	10 to 20 minutes
Environment	Area with room enough to roll or throw balls
Materials	Several balloons and balls of various sizes, textures, and colors

Benefits

physical: large muscle use, range of motion, hand-eye coordination

cognitive: discriminating visually, concentrating, describing, naming, selecting

emotional: enjoyment, happiness, excitement, surprise, pleasure, caution

social: interacting with objects, interacting with others

Activity

- Blow up two or three balloons of different colors. Encourage the resident to help if able.
  - Ask the resident which is his or her favorite color.
  - Ask him/her to touch the balloon which is his/her favorite color.
  - Encourage the resident to handle the balloon and throw it to you.
  - Ask the resident if s/he would like to pop the balloon.
- Show the resident several balls of various shapes, textures, and colors.
  - Identify the games these balls are used with—i.e. football, basketball, baseball.
  - Roll or throw the balls to the resident.
  - Encourage the resident to handle the balls.

Conversation Starters

- Talk about occasions where balloons have been used in the resident's life or when they are used in the facility.
- Talk about community little league, school teams, etc.
- Talk about the games the resident played in childhood that required a ball.

Ball Darts

Group Size	One on one or small group
Time	10 to 15 minutes
Environment	Wall space approximately five feet wide by five feet high
Materials	Thin piece of 1/4 inch plywood measuring 4 1/2 feet by 3 1/2 feet
	Special fabric that Velcro will attach to, of same measurement as above, tacked to board
	Velcro balls of different colors
	One black broad tipped marker to mark scores on target

Benefits

physical: upper body range of motion, fine motor manipulation, eye-hand coordination

cognitive: math skills, motor planning, following directions, distinguishing, identifying, calculating

emotional: spirit of competition, enjoyment, satisfaction, happiness, excitement, enthusiasm, pride

social: interaction with objects, interaction with others

Activity

Ask the resident to throw the Velcro ball at the target. Scores may be recorded to determine a winner or contestants may vie to see who gets closest to the center.

Conversation Starters

- Did you ever play darts when you were young? Where did you play? Who did you play with?
- What kind of sports have you played?

Pass the Ball

Group Size	One on one or small group
Time	5 to 10 minutes
Environment	Uncluttered space of five to ten feet that will allow some throwing, catching and bouncing
Materials	Tennis ball, beach ball, punch ball, nerf ball, wiffle ball, baseball, etc.

Benefits

physical: eye-hand coordination, upper body range of motion, fine motor manipulation

cognitive: concentrating, following directions, sequencing, distinguishing, describing, identifying, matching

emotional: feelings of joy and satisfaction from successfully throwing and catching the ball

social: interacting with others, interacting with objects, reacting to objects

Activity

- Pass the balls, one by one, to each resident. Have him/her squeeze each ball with one or two hands then have the resident pass it to the next person. As the ball is being passed, talk about how it feels. Is it easy or hard to squeeze? What types of games have you played with this ball?
- Bounce punch ball. Throw and catch other balls back and forth.
- For those with severe dementia, limit to one ball and one activity at a time.

Conversation Starters

- Do you recognize any of these balls?
- What kind of games or sports are played with these balls? (Show volleyball, tennis ball, football, soccer ball, jacks ball, beach ball, etc.)

Exercises Using Elastic

Group Size	Small group
Time	10 to 15 minutes
Environment	May be done in room or activity area
Materials	Long piece of 1 inch elastic sewed together to make a circle; tape of slow instrumental music, tape player

Benefits

physical: large muscle movement, full range of motion, upper body range of motion

cognitive: concentrating, following the leader, distinguishing, matching, reproducing

emotional: satisfaction of working together with others, joy of moving body to music

social: interacting with objects, reacting to objects, reacting to others

spiritual: feeling connected to others, sense of belonging to a group

Activity

- Arrange the room so that everyone is sitting in a circle.
- Ask each person to hold onto the elastic with both hands.
- As the music begins, lead the residents through different stretching movements, using the elastic as a connector between people.
- This activity is helpful to those who cannot normally follow someone leading exercises. Holding onto the elastic aids the person along, giving him/her support where needed.

Conversation Starters

- What does the elastic remind you of?
- Have you ever made something that required an elastic waist band? Tell me about it.
- What other uses can you think of for elastic?

Blowing

Group Size	One on one
Time	10 to 15 minutes
Environment	Quiet area with table and chairs
Materials	Matches, candle, feather, Ping-Pong ball, bubble solution
Warning	*Do not* use open flame near oxygen and only with the permission of the Director of Nursing Services

Benefits

physical: fine motor control of facial muscles, exercising respiratory capacity

cognitive: concentrating, following directions, reproducing, describing, giving examples

emotional: enjoyment, sense of accomplishment, surprise

social: interacting with others, interacting with objects, reacting to objects

Activity

- Using one item at a time, demonstrate blowing and then encourage the resident to try.
- *Match:* light the match and then blow it out.
- *Candle:* light the candle, then blow it out.
- *Feather:* Hold the feather in front of the mouth and gently blow. Observe the parts of the feather as it is blown. Put the feather on the table and blow it across the surface.
- *Ping-Pong ball:* Place the Ping-Pong ball on the table and blow it to the other side.
- *Bubble solution:* Blow bubbles—make small and large bubbles.

Conversation Starters

- What kind of matches have you used?
- What occasions do we use candles for?
- Where do we usually find feathers?
- What do the bubbles make you think of?

Ribbon Dance

Group Size	Small group
Time	15 to 20 minutes
Environment	Activity room, with space to dance around in a small circle. Linoleum or wooden floor is preferred
Materials	Music: waltz, fox trot, any music with a moderate beat. For dancing: scarves, long ribbon that will reach around the entire circle

Benefits

physical: large muscle range of motion, cardiovascular endurance

cognitive: concentrating, sequencing movements, following directions, moving in rhythm

emotional: joy, satisfaction of moving to music, excitement, peacefulness, pride

social: interacting with others, reacting to objects, interacting with objects

Activity

- Have chairs arranged in a circle before residents arrive. Introduce activity by stating that dancing is any movement to music.

- Put on music with a moderate, strong beat and let residents clap and sway to the music. Make up a sequence of two combined movements sitting in chairs and have residents copy your movements. Add additional movements one at a time, according to the ability level of residents.

- Hand out long ribbon so that everyone is holding it in the circle. Now lead them together in movements such as raising both hands and swaying to the right and left. Put music on and let them move to the music.

Conversation Starters

- What kinds of music did you dance to when you were younger?

- How does the music make you feel?
- Do you have someone you especially like to dance with?

Scarf Dance

<table>
<tr><td>**Group Size**</td><td>Small group</td></tr>
<tr><td>**Time**</td><td>15 to 20 minutes</td></tr>
<tr><td>**Environment**</td><td>Open space to allow for freedom of movement; wooden or linoleum floor preferred</td></tr>
<tr><td>**Materials**</td><td>A variety of colored scarves, one for each person
Music with a moderate beat</td></tr>
</table>

Benefits

physical: large muscle movement, cardiovascular endurance, upper body range of motion

cognitive: concentrating, remembering, sequencing, matching movements of others, describing, modifying, creating

emotional: joy, satisfaction of moving to music, peacefulness, enthusiasm

social: interacting with others, interacting with objects

Activity

- Start with everyone sitting in a circle. Put easy, moderate beat music on and lead residents through different arm movements using scarves as a warm up.
- Arrange residents in partners (if possible one mobile partner with one sitting in a chair). Put on waltz (3/4 time) or fox trot (4/4 time) music and demonstrate movements possible with the scarves.
- Let them create their own movements, each holding on to one end of the scarf. The residents who are more able can twirl under the scarf and go around the chair lifting the scarf over the resident in the chair.

Conversation Starters

- What colors are the scarves?
- What kind of scarves did you wear?
- Can you think of any other ways to use scarves?
- What kind of music do you like?
- How does this music make you feel?

Stretching Exercises

Group Size	One on one
Time	15 to 20 minutes
Environment	Circle of straight backed chairs
Materials	Slow music (optional), chairs

Benefits

physical: range of motion, basic motor movements, body awareness, cardiovascular endurance

cognitive: concentrating, creating, following directions

emotional: satisfaction, relief, excitement, peacefulness, enthusiasm, pride, confidence

social: self-concept, reaction to others

Activity

- *Leg and ankles:* raise knee, and extend leg forward; slowly lower leg. Circle ankles clockwise, then counterclockwise; toes up, toes down, in and out.
- *Modified half-spinal twist:* twist torso to right; looking over right shoulder as far as comfortable; repeat to left
- *Side stretch:* arms at side; bend at waist to right; back to starting position; left; slow, smooth motion
- *Hand and arm:* make a fist, then relax. Circle wrists clockwise, then counterclockwise. Shrug shoulders up and down, circle elbow around clockwise, then counterclockwise.
- *Neck:* move head slowly up and down; then side to side. Move head in semi-circular action.
- *Ending:* gently move each joint through a comfortable range-of-motion.

Conversation Starters

- How does it feel to stretch?
- When do you usually stretch during the day?
- Who do you know that does exercises?
- What other ways do you exercise?

Note: Be careful not to tilt the head back, as it may pinch nerves in the vertebrae. Also, do not make full circles with the head, as this may lead to dizziness.

The Parachute

Group Size	Small group
Time	10 to 15 minutes
Environment	Space large enough for a parachute to be stretched out and people seated around the perimeter
Materials	Parachute (may use sheet, tablecloth, or material from old umbrella)
	Nerf balls and balloons
	Record or tape of music (may use lively or slow music depending of the physical capabilities of the residents)

Benefits

physical: enhance arm, hand, shoulder, and upper body strength and upper body range of motion; stimulate hand-eye coordination

cognitive: concentrating, creating, estimating, predicting, sequencing movements

emotional: feelings of satisfaction in doing physical activity, joy, excitement, enthusiasm

social: interacting with others, reacting to objects, reacting to others

Activity

- Ask the residents to hold the edge of the parachute. Tell them that everyone is to lift the parachute up over their heads on the count of three. The parachute will catch the air underneath and mushroom out at the peak of its height. Still holding on, allow the material to slowly float down. Repeat several times. This part of the activity can be done to music. Break activity into short periods of two or three minutes to avoid fatigue.
- Popcorn: Place a few nerf balls on the taut material and ask the residents to bounce the balls by rapidly moving the material up and down.
- See if everyone can work together to roll one ball all the way around the parachute.

**Conversation
Starters**

- What do you feel when we lift the parachute? Do you feel the breeze?
- What else could we do with the parachute?

Reaching the Top Shelf

Group Size	One on one
Time	5 to 20 minutes
Environment	Wall space with two or three shelves or a portable shelf unit with wheels that can be locked. Shelves should be at face level and above.
Materials	Shelves Soft, colorful, items such as small toy animals, cloth blocks, hats, or small books

Benefits

physical: stretching, tactile stimulation, fine motor manipulation

cognitive: concentrating, describing, identifying, problem solving

emotional: sense of accomplishment, happiness, pride

social: interacting with others, interacting with objects

Activity

Ask the resident to take items from the shelves one at a time. Discuss each item and then return it to the shelf.

Conversation Starters

- Tell me about this item.
- Did you have shelves you couldn't reach?
- How did you get items from those shelves?

Reaching for Texture

Group Size	One on one
Time	5 to 15 minutes
Environment	Area with wall space for hangings
Materials	Wall hangings made of carpet samples in different colors and textures

Benefits

physical: stretching, tactile stimulation, range of motion, fine motor manipulation

cognitive: concentrating, identifying, describing, matching, differentiating

emotional: enjoyment of tactile feelings

Activity

- Arrange two or three wall hangings near each other at different heights. Encourage the resident to feel the hangings, exploring the different textures and colors.
- Note: the residents will often return to this activity on their own, once they are introduced to it several times.

Conversation Starters

- How does this feel to you?
- Does this wall hanging remind you of anything?
- Did you have carpeting in your home? What color was it?
- How did you clean your rugs when you were young?

Reach for the Gold

Group Size	One on one
Time	5 to 15 minutes
Environment	Wall space for measuring stick
Materials	Measuring stick mounted on wall or numbers painted on the wall
	Circle of gold at the top of the measure

Benefits

physical: flexion, range of motion

cognitive: concentrating, identifying, counting, following directions

emotional: feeling of accomplishment

social: reaction to objects, interactions with others

Activity

- Demonstrate starting at the bottom of the measuring stick and climbing with hands toward the top. Encourage the resident to slowly climb the measure while counting the numbers. When s/he reaches the gold circle give a reward such as a gold ribbon.
- Note: climbing slowly gives a better stretch.
- You might use the resident's favorite color instead of the gold.

Conversation Starters

- How does it feel to stretch?
- When do you usually stretch?
- Do you like gold?
- What things can you think of that are gold?

Chapter 14

Sensory Stimulation

Sensory stimulation is important to the adult who's impaired. This kind of activity helps to maintain the senses of hearing, vision, touch, smell, and taste. These senses are essential to keep in touch with one's world. Our awareness of reality depends on our senses. The adult who is cognitively impaired may have little response to his/her surroundings. We need to continue to encourage whatever awareness there is by stimulating his/her senses.

Whenever possible, exercise (stimulate) as many senses as possible. Start with hearing by describing or explaining, then vision by providing an item or picture for the resident to see. Next encourage the resident to touch or to hold the item. Encourage smelling and end the activity with taste when appropriate.

These activities are intended to give you ideas for sensory activities you can use. Your knowledge of the resident and your imagination will enlarge the scope of activities.

Hand Massage

Group Size	One on one
Time	5 to 15 minutes
Environment	Individual's room
Materials	Mineral oil, scented oil, or hand lotion

Benefits

physical: improves circulation in hands and arms and lubricates dry skin

cognitive: relaxes mind and body

emotional: feelings of comfort and security are evoked

social: reacting to others, interacting with others

Activity

- Rub oil on hands and arms, using gentle, rubbing strokes. Always rub arm upwards toward the heart to help increase circulation of blood.
- During the massage, attempt conversation with the individual by talking about familiar things.

Conversation Starters

- Tell me about your family. (Ask about specific family members, especially about family achievements or celebrations.)
- Note any cards displayed. Ask about the people who sent them.
- What things did you do to help you feel pampered? (Hair care, manicures or pedicures, massage, steam baths, etc.)

Note: If the resident has cracked skin or open sores, please do not touch that area. Find another area of the body that will not offend the resident (perhaps the feet or forehead). As always wash hands thoroughly after any touching activity.

Sound Effects

Group Size	One on one
Time	5 to 10 minutes
Environment	Quiet room with comfortable chair
Materials	Records or tapes of sound effects such as:
	Ocean waves, fire crackling, baby crying, dog barking, water faucet running, kids laughing, waterfalls, teakettle whistling
	Tapes may be found at libraries and college theater departments, or tape your own sounds

Benefits

cognitive: stimulates mind to remember sounds
emotional: expression of feelings associated with sounds
social: reaction to objects (sounds)

Activity

- Make the resident comfortable and then play the record or tape. Ask the resident to identify the sound. Possibly the sound will bring back memories that could stimulate the resident to verbalize some feelings. Individuals who are disoriented may not be able to verbalize, but still may enjoy listening and identifying the sounds.
- Residents with dementia may be unable to distinguish taped sounds from reality. They may become agitated thinking the sounds are real. Use non-threatening sounds (such as kids laughing or birds singing) with these individuals and cease activity if agitation is noted.

Conversation Starters

- What sounds do you hear?
- Are these sounds familiar to you?
- What memories do these sounds bring to you?

Touching Exercises

Group Size	One on one
Time	5 to 10 minutes
Environment	Quiet area with comfortable chairs
Materials	A variety of items that have unique textures:
	A blotter, cork, corn silk husk, candle, emery board, peeled hard cooked egg, flower, ice, Jell-O (made with half the water called for in directions), moss, powder puff, raw potato that has been half peeled, rabbit's foot, rope, rubber toy animal, rubber glove filled with sand, sawdust, velvet, silk, sponge

Benefits

physical: tactile stimulation
cognitive: recognizing objects, discriminating textures
emotional: evoke feelings associated with textures
social: interacting with objects, reacting to objects

Activity

- Give the resident a variety of objects to feel, one at a time. Limit number of objects to 4 or 5 each session.
- Encourage the resident to talk about the texture of the object.
- For the resident who is disoriented you might use just edible objects and include the sense of taste in the experience.

Conversation Starters

- What does this object feel like?
- Can you think of something else that feels similar to this?
- What kinds of things do you like to touch and handle?

Note: Make sure that any food you serve the residents is allowed by his/her physician's current orders regarding food, calorie intake, and consistency. Record all food eaten if that is appropriate.

Smelling

Group Size	One on one
Time	5 to 10 minutes
Environment	Quiet area with table and chairs
Materials	Small bottles with contents of brown sugar, coffee, tea, pepper, tobacco, candy, soap, face powder, perfume, vinegar, vanilla, almond, lemon, apple, banana, nutmeg, cloves, rum, sherry

Benefits

cognitive: recognizing, describing, matching, giving examples

emotional: evokes emotions associated with smells

social: interacting with others, reacting to objects

Activity

• Ask the individual to sniff one bottle at a time without looking into the contents and identify the scent. Limit the number to 4 to 6 per session.

• Encourage the individual to talk about the memories evoked.

Conversation Starters

• How would you rate your sense of smell?

• Was there a time in your life when you had an especially acute sense of smell?

• What smells do you remember from your childhood? From your teens? From adulthood?

• Could you recognize your home (or school, or church, or work place) by its smell?

Tea Tasting

Group Size	One on one
Time	10 to 15 minutes
Environment	Table with space to display several different flavors of tea
Materials	Boxes of different flavored tea Cups of prepared tea

Benefits

physical: stimulate sense of taste

cognitive: distinguishing among the different flavors

emotional: provide opportunity for individual to feel successful

social: interacting with others, reacting to objects

spiritual: acceptance of self

Activity

- Present the individual with boxes of tea with pictures of the fruit on the box. Let him/her look at the pictures and smell the aroma of the tea. Talk about the different flavors.
- Demonstrate by tasting some of the brewed tea. Then say what flavor you tasted and point to the picture on the appropriate box. Allow the person to choose a cup and taste the tea. Help him/her to identify the flavor.

Conversation Starters

- Have you ever had herbal teas? What kind have you tried? Which one did you like best?
- Do you associate tea drinking with any special occasion? (For instance when you were sick or when there were special visitors.)
- Did you use tea bags or loose tea?
- Did you use the used tea leaves in any way? (For instance, in the garden or to tint fabric.)

Note: Make sure that anything you serve the resident is allowed by his/her physician's current orders regarding food, calorie intake, and consistency. Record all food eaten if that is appropriate.

Fruit Flavors

Group Size	One on one
Time	10 to 15 minutes
Environment	Table and chairs
Materials	Three or four pieces of fruit
	Slices of the same fruit cut up and placed in separate bowls

Benefits

physical: stimulates sense of taste
cognitive: remembering the taste of different fruits
emotional: feelings of success
social: interaction with others

Activity

- Encourage the resident to look at and handle the whole fruit while you name the fruit.
- Demonstrate for the resident by tasting one of the slices of the fruit and saying the name or the fruit, then selecting the corresponding whole fruit. Then ask the resident to taste a slice and select the fruit, too.
- Reward participation with verbal encouragement.

Conversation Starters

- What is your favorite fruit?
- What do you think the saying "an apple a day keeps the doctor away" means?
- What special occasions do you associate with fruit? (For instance, fruit in stockings at Christmas, or apples at Halloween.)

Note: Make sure that anything you serve the resident is allowed by his/her physician's current orders regarding food, calorie intake, and consistency. Record all food eaten if that is appropriate.

Vegetables

Group Size	One on one
Time	10 to 20 minutes
Environment	Area with table and chairs—kitchen setting
Materials	Fresh vegetables from local market or garden
	2 ears of corn, 5 new potatoes, green beans, onion

Benefits

physical: fine motor manipulation, hand-eye coordination

cognitive: defining, describing, distinguishing, naming, giving examples

emotional: pleasure, satisfaction, joy, happiness, pride, pleasure, contentment

social: interacting with others, reacting to objects

Activity

- Pull each vegetable out of the bag one at a time. Let the resident look at it, feet it, smell it.
- Encourage the resident to talk about each vegetable. Ask the resident to show you how s/he would prepare the vegetable for cooking.
- Stick a fork in the onion and allow the juice to be smelled. Ask for memories of eyes watering when peeling or slicing onions.
- With the resident who is more able, you could have him/her help peel and slice the vegetables, put them in a pan, and cook them. If allowed, let the resident eat the vegetables for his/her dinner.

Conversation Starters

- What are different ways you can fix corn (potatoes, beans, etc.)?
- Do you remember a special time when you and your family ate corn?
- Did you grow and or can your own vegetables? Tell me about your garden. About canning.

Note: Make sure that anything you serve the resident is allowed by his/her physician's current orders regarding food, calorie intake, and consistency. Record all food eaten if that is appropriate.

Remembering Hand Muffs

Group Size	One on one
Time	10 to 15 minutes
Environment	Quiet space
Materials	Old fur hand muff

Benefits

physical: fine motor manipulation, tactile stimulation

cognitive: describing, defining, distinguishing, explaining, giving examples

emotional: calm, comforting effects of stroking and cuddling fur

social: interacting with others, reacting to objects

Activity

- Allow the resident to feel and try on the muff.
- Ask the resident to describe the muff and tell about the memories it brings.
- Stroke the fur and discuss how it feels.

Conversation Starters

- Did you ever wear a muff? Where did you wear it?
- Did it serve its purpose or was it simply for fashion?
- What was your muff made of?
- What was it like on the inside? On the outside?
- Does this fur feel like the fur of a pet you once had?
- What other clothing did you have that had fur on it?

Textured Materials

Group Size	One on one
Time	5 to 15 minutes
Environment	Quiet area with comfortable chairs
Materials	Audio tape of soothing music or nature sounds
	Small pieces of material of different textures such as:
	Velvet, corduroy, wool, fur, cotton, leather, satin, flannel, silk

Benefits

physical: tactile stimulation
cognitive: describing, distinguishing
emotional: enjoyment, peacefulness
social: interacting with others, reacting to objects

Activity

- With background music playing softly, gently rub each piece of material on the resident's arm
- Encourage the resident to feel each piece. Discuss the material: color, texture, etc.

Conversation Starters

- How does this material feel?
- What does this material make you think of?
- Would this be a material you would like to wear?
- Do you see anything in this room that is the same color as this material?

Body Sense

Group Size	One on one
Time	10 to 20 minutes
Environment	The resident's room, quiet, with no distractions
Materials	None needed

Benefits

physical: tactile stimulation, gentle range of motion
cognitive: distinguishing, identifying, explaining
social: interaction with another

Activity

- Make the resident comfortable in bed. Starting with the head, encourage the resident to touch specific areas of his/her body and talk about them. If the resident is unable to follow directions, gently help him/her to touch.
- *Head:* Touch the person's hair; talk about the color, texture, and any other distinguishing features. Encourage the resident to touch his/her hair. Touch the persons eyes; talk about the color and some of the things the person is seeing. Do the same with the mouth, encouraging the person to touch.
- *Hands:* Touch the hands and talk about the work those hands have done. Encourage the person to stroke his/her hands.
- *Feet:* Touch the feet and talk about where those feet have been.
- *Chest:* Touch the chest over the heart. Talk about the loves of the person.
- *Stomach:* Touch the stomach and talk about the foods the person has eaten or the hungers s/he has experienced.

Conversation Starters

- Use the touch and the part of the body to guide conversation. Even if the resident is unable to talk, your comments will be meaningful.

Note: If the resident has cracked skin or open sores, please do not touch that area. Touch areas of the body that will not offend the resident.

Visual Stimulation

Group Size	One on one
Time	10 to 15 minutes
Environment	Quiet place with good light and minimal visual distractions
Materials	Primary colors and patterns (stripes, checks, etc.) attached to 8½ x 11 pieces of cardboard

Benefits

cognitive: concentrating, identifying, matching, selecting
emotional: joy in seeing colors
social: interacting with others, reacting to objects

Activity

- Hold a color or pattern card in front of the resident.
- Name the color or pattern.
- Encourage the resident to touch the card.
- Point out other things in the room or on clothing that are the same color.
- Use only one color at a time and spend several minutes on each color.
- You may wish to use only one color per session.

Conversation Starters

- Do you have a favorite color?
- Do you like patterns? Can you see something in the room that has a similar pattern?

Sound Stimulation

Group Size	One on one
Time	10 to 15 minutes
Environment	Quiet place with no distractions
Materials	Bell, cellophane, tuning fork, pitch pipe, or harmonica

Benefits

cognitive: distinguishing, selecting, changing direction
emotional: enjoyment of sounds
social: reacting to others, reacting to objects

Activity

- Make the resident comfortable in a chair or bed.
- Using one sound instrument at a time, make the sound in front of the resident and discuss how it sounds.
- Move the sound to the right side of the head and repeat the sound.
- Note any tendency to turn the head. Repeat on the other side of the head.
- Repeat the exercise with one instrument several times. You may want to use only one sound during a session or you may try two or three.
- Stop the activity at any sign of agitation.

Conversation Starters

- See the bell? What kind of sound does the bell make?
- Listen to the bell sound. Does the sound of the bell remind you of anything?
- Where is the bell now (when ringing at the side of the head)?
- Repeat with other sounds.

Stress Relief

Group Size	One on one
Time	5 to 15 minutes
Environment	Can be used anywhere
Materials	Heavy duty balloon partially filled with sand

Benefits

physical: upper body range of motion, fine motor manipulation

cognitive: soothing from repetitive motion, distinguishing, reproducing

emotional: enjoyment of kneading with hand

social: reacting to objects, interacting with objects, interacting with others

Activity

- Check the balloon to be sure there are no holes and the neck is securely tied.
- Demonstrate by kneading the balloon in your hands.
- Give the balloon to the resident and gently help him/her to knead it.

Conversation Starters

- What does this feel like?
- Can you make shapes with the balloon?
- What other things does one knead?

Rocking Chair

Group Size	One on one
Time	10 to 15 minutes
Environment	Quiet area with space for a rocking chair
Materials	Rocking chairs Record, CD, or tape of music with strong rhythm

Benefits

physical: relaxation of tense muscles, strength and flexion, stimulation of inner ear

cognitive: concentrating, following directions, describing

emotional: enjoyment of rhythmic activity

social: interacting with objects (rocking chair), interacting with others

Activity

- Place the resident in a rocking chair facing you. Start the music and begin rocking to the music.
- Encourage the resident to follow your lead in raising and lowering legs, kicking feet, clapping hands, moving shoulders, arms, and hands.
- Encourage relaxation by smiling. One might even sing along with the music.

Conversation Starters

- What do you like about rocking?
- When have you used a rocking chair?
- Tell me about your favorite rocking chair.

Plastic Bag Painting

Group Size	One on one
Time	10 to 15 minutes
Environment	Table with space to place a few plastic bags
Materials	Quart size zip lock bags (7" x 8") Finger paint set with 6 colors

Benefits

physical: fine motor coordination: good for arthritic hands

cognitive: identifying color, matching action to memories

emotional: enjoyment, happiness, satisfaction, contentment, feelings of success

social: interacting with objects, interacting with others

Activity

- Place approximately one large teaspoon of each color paint in a bag. Do not mix the colors, let the resident do that.
- Make sure the bag has no air trapped inside and seal the zip lock opening.
- Present the resident with the plastic bags filled with paints. Let him/her look at the bags. Talk about the different colors that are present in the bags.
- Demonstrate painting by taking hands and fingers and moving the different colored paint inside the bag to make unique designs and integrated colors.
- Ask the resident to take a bag and do the same.

Conversation Starters

- Have you ever finger painted? What kind of paper did you use? Did you every do it this way with plastic bags?
- Do you associate this activity with any special occasion? Do you have a story to tell about finger painting or any kind of painting?
- Who did you paint with? Where did you paint?